Resistance to Targeted Anti-Cancer Therapeutics

Volume 13

Series Editor:
Benjamin Bonavida

More information about this series at http://www.springer.com/series/11727

Augusto Villanueva
Editor

Resistance to Molecular Therapies for Hepatocellular Carcinoma

Springer

Editor
Augusto Villanueva
Division of Liver Diseases
Tisch Cancer Institute
Icahn School of Medicine at Mount Sinai
Graduate School of Biomedical Sciences
New York, NY, USA

ISSN 2196-5501 ISSN 2196-551X (electronic)
Resistance to Targeted Anti-Cancer Therapeutics
ISBN 978-3-319-56196-7 ISBN 978-3-319-56197-4 (eBook)
DOI 10.1007/978-3-319-56197-4

Library of Congress Control Number: 2017943130

Printed on acid-free paper

This Springer imprint is published by Springer Nature
The registered company is Springer International Publishing AG
The registered company address is: Gewerbestrasse 11, 6330 Cham, Switzerland

This volume is dedicated to Susana and our little Emma.

“Resistance to Targeted Anti-Cancer Therapeutics”: Aims and Scope

For several decades, treatment of cancer consisted of chemotherapeutic drugs, radiation, and hormonal therapies. Those were not tumor specific and exhibited several toxicities. During the last several years, targeted cancer therapies (molecularly targeted drugs) have been developed, consisting of immunotherapies (cell mediated and antibody), drugs, or biologicals that can block the growth and spread of cancer by interfering with surface receptors and with specific dysregulated gene products that control tumor cell growth and progression. These include several FDA-approved drugs/antibodies/inhibitors that interfere with cell growth signaling or tumor blood vessel development, promote the cell death of cancer cells, stimulate the immune system to destroy specific cancer cells, and deliver toxic drugs to cancer cells. Targeted cancer therapies are being used alone or in combination with conventional drugs and other targeted therapies.

One of the major problems that arise following treatment with both conventional therapies and targeted cancer therapies is the development of resistance, preexisting in a subset of cancer cells or cancer stem cells and/or induced by the treatments. Tumor cell resistance to targeted therapies remains a major hurdle, and, therefore, several strategies are being considered in delineating the underlining molecular mechanisms of resistance and the development of novel drugs to reverse both the innate and acquired resistance to various targeted therapeutic regimens.

The new series *Resistance to Targeted Anti-Cancer Therapeutics* was inaugurated and focuses on the clinical application of targeted cancer therapies (either approved by the FDA or in clinical trials) and the resistance observed by these therapies. Each book will consist of updated reviews on a specific target therapeutic and strategies to overcome resistance at the biochemical, molecular, and both genetic and epigenetic levels. This new series is timely and should be of significant interest to clinicians, scientists, trainees, students, and pharmaceutical companies.

Benjamin Bonavida
David Geffen School of Medicine at UCLA
University of California, Los Angeles
Los Angeles, CA, 90025, USA

About the Editor

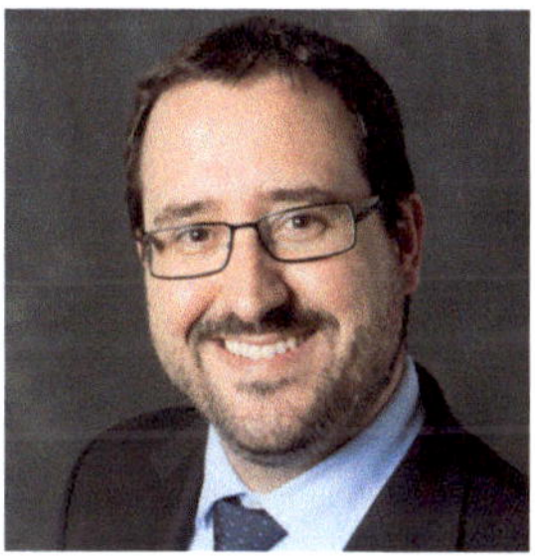

Augusto Villanueva is an Assistant Professor at the Division of Liver Diseases of the Icahn School of Medicine at Mount Sinai (New York). He received his medical degree from the University of Santiago de Compostela (Spain), achieving the National Award for Excellence in Academic Performance. After completing his residency of Gastroenterology and Hepatology in 2005, he joined the Division of Liver Diseases at Mount Sinai School of Medicine (New York), where he conducted extensive research in different translational aspects of liver cancer including molecular-based classification and prognosis prediction (i.e., gene signatures), integrative genomic analyses, and characterization of deregulated signaling pathways as novel therapeutic targets. In 2008, Dr. Villanueva obtained a Ph.D. degree from the University of Santiago de Compostela on Biomedical Sciences. Later, he received a Sheila Sherlock fellowship from the European Association for the Study of the Liver and moved to the Liver Cancer Translational Research Laboratory of the BCLC Group, Hospital Clinic, Barcelona (Spain). In 2010, he became the scientific manager of the HEPTROMIC consortium, one of the first consortia funded by the European Commission (FP7 program) focused on liver cancer research. In early 2013, he joined the Institute of Liver Studies at King's College Hospital (London, UK), as Senior Lecturer and Consultant Hepatologist. Since 2014, he works at the Liver Cancer Program (Icahn School of Medicine at Mount Sinai, New York) where he is developing projects related to mechanisms of liver cancer evolution and treatment resistance. He is also interested in using minimally invasive tools to generate novel prognostic and predictive biomarkers (i.e., liquid biopsy). Dr. Villanueva has more than 85 peer-reviewed publications (6,950 citations, H-index 37) including articles in *The New England Journal of Medicine*, *Nature Genetics*, *Nature Biotechnology*, *Journal of Clinical Investigation*, *Gastroenterology*, *Hepatology*, *Cancer Research*, and *Journal of*

Hepatology, among others. He wrote more than 10 book chapters and serves as Associate Editor for the *Journal of Hepatology* and *Liver Cancer*. He has received numerous awards including the *Rising Star Gastroenterologist* from the United European Gastroenterology and the *Alan Hofmann Clinical and Translational Award* from the American Association for the Study for Liver Diseases.

Preface

Liver cancer has emerged as a major health problem. Unlike most human malignancies, its incidence and mortality has increased in the last 30 years. Indeed, the 2016 report from the US National Cancer Institute warns about this negative trend in liver cancer mortality. The treatment of liver cancer changed significantly in 2007. The landmark SHARP trial demonstrated how sorafenib increases survival in liver cancer patients, without inducing major drug toxicity. Survival benefits reached 3 months on average, but ultimately, most patients progressed. Since then, numerous clinical trials have tried to improve or parallel the results achieved with sorafenib, but with very limited success. It was not until 2016 when regorafenib showed its ability to extend survival in patients who progressed to sorafenib. This represents the first effective second-line therapy for liver cancer patients, which establishes a new milestone in the treatment of this disease. Despite this improvement, most tumors become resistant, and ultimately patients succumb to the disease.

The primary aim of this book is to provide a multidimensional evaluation of the mechanisms and consequences of treatment resistance in liver cancer. We have gathered a set of worldwide experts to approach this complex problem from different angles, including molecular heterogeneity, cancer stem cell biology, and the role of the tumor microenvironment, with a particular focus on the immune system. Now that systemic therapies are improving outcomes in liver cancer patients, the importance of understanding mechanisms of resistance cannot be overemphasized. Clearly, leveraging on this knowledge is the best way to improve drug design and move toward a definitive cure.

New York, NY, USA | Augusto Villanueva

Contents

Tumor Heterogeneity and Resistance to Targeted Therapies in Hepatocellular Carcinoma

Amanda J. Craig, Ismail Labgaa, Carlos Villacorta-Martin, Massih Ningarhari, and Augusto Villanueva

Abstract Hepatocellular carcinoma is a heterogeneous disease, both phenotypically and genetically. This heterogeneity can be observed over a spectrum ranging among tumors of different patients, multiple nodules of one patient and even within a single tumor nodule. As demonstrated in other tumor types, this diversity may contribute to the development of drug resistance. The mechanisms behind intratumoral heterogeneity are not yet fully understood, and potential theories include the clonal evolution or cancer stem cells differentiation hierarchy. In recent years, many technologies have helped assess clonal content of tumors, including multiregional and single cell next generation sequencing. Changes in clonal content over time and during treatment can now be easily tracked, which will provide novel

A.J. Craig • C. Villacorta-Martin
Liver Cancer Program, Division of Liver Diseases, Tisch Cancer Institute, Department of Medicine, Graduate School of Biomedical Sciences, Icahn School of Medicine at Mount Sinai, New York, NY, USA

I. Labgaa
Division of Visceral Surgery, Lausanne University Hospital CHUV, Lausanne, Switzerland

Liver Cancer Program, Division of Liver Diseases, Tisch Cancer Institute, Department of Medicine, Graduate School of Biomedical Sciences, Icahn School of Medicine at Mount Sinai, New York, NY, USA

M. Ningarhari
CHRU Lille, Hôpital Huriez, Service des Maladies de l'Appareil Digestif et de la Nutrition, Inserm, LIRIC-UMR995, Univ Lille, Lille, France

A. Villanueva (✉)
Liver Cancer Program, Division of Liver Diseases, Tisch Cancer Institute, Department of Medicine, Graduate School of Biomedical Sciences, Icahn School of Medicine at Mount Sinai, New York, NY, USA

Division of Hematology and Medical Oncology, Department of Medicine, Icahn School of Medicine at Mount Sinai, New York, NY, USA
e-mail: augusto.villanueva@mssm.edu

A. Villanueva (ed.), *Resistance to Molecular Therapies for Hepatocellular Carcinoma*, Resistance to Targeted Anti-Cancer Therapeutics,
DOI 10.1007/978-3-319-56197-4_1

insights into cancer evolution and mechanisms of treatment resistance. This will be critical to provide novel therapeutic targets for second and third line therapies in hepatocellular carcinoma.

Keywords Biomarker • Cancer evolution • Clonality • Intra-tumor heterogeneity • Liquid biopsy

Abbreviations

18F-FDG	Fludeoxy-glucose
AFP	Alpha-fetoprotein
BEAMing	Beads, emulsion, amplification, and magnetics
cfDNA	Cell free DNA
CGH	Comparative genomic hybridization
CNA	Copy number alteration
CNV	Copy number variation
CSCs	Cancer stem cells
CT	Computed tomography
CTC	Circulating tumor cells
ctDNA	Circulating tumor DNA
EMT	Epithelial to mesenchymal transition
EpCAM	Epithelial cell adhesion molecule
FACS	Fluorescence-activated cell sorting
GS	Glutamine synthetase
HBV	Hepatitis B virus
HCC	Hepatocellular carcinoma
HCV	Hepatitis C virus
IHC	Immunohistochemistry
mCRC	Metastatic colorectal cancer
MDS	Multidimensional scaling
MRI	Magnetic resonance imaging
NGS	Next generation sequencing
nmCRC	Nonmetastatic colorectal cancer
PCA	Principle component analysis
PDX	Patient derived xenograft
PET	Positron emission tomography
RFLP	Restriction fragment length polymorphism
SNV	Single nucleotide variants
SSCP	Single-strand conformation polymorphism
TACE	Trans-arterial chemoembolization

Introduction

Molecular heterogeneity in cancer can be defined as the distinct genetic alterations and phenotypes among cancer cells, found either between patients or within the same (i.e., intra-tumor) or multiple (i.e., inter-tumor) nodules originating from the same patient [1]. In regards to intra-tumor heterogeneity, the distinctions among cancer cells are demonstrated by the presence of numerous sub-clones within a single tumor mass. A sub-clone is defined as any cell population with a mutation cell fraction less than 1 [2], or in other words, a mutation that is not present in all cells. Those mutations that give a fitness advantage to that sub-clone over others will lead to an outgrowth. Notably, not all acquired mutations create a phenotype with a fitness advantage. These mutations accumulate throughout the tumor evolution and are considered passenger events [2].

Several theories have been proposed as to how intra-tumor heterogeneity develops (Table 1). The first is clonal evolution, which was initially proposed by Peter Nowell in 1976 [3]. This theory suggests that cancer cells acquire mutations over time, some of which provide a gain of fitness. Cells that acquire mutations that increase their fitness will become the dominant clone within the tumor. This competition occurs throughout the lifetime of a tumor, resulting in either linear or branched evolution patterns. Tumors that follow a branched evolution trajectory will develop numerous sub-clones with distinct genetic profiles. Another theory describes cancer stem cells (CSCs) as the cause of intra-tumor heterogeneity [4]. CSCs are proposed to be cells with unlimited self-renewal capabilities, which can ultimately give rise to the various clones found within the tumor. A third model describing intra-tumor heterogeneity is neutral evolution [5]. This model suggests that there is no competition between tumor clones. A mutational load that is proportional to the proliferation and mutation rates of the tumor characterizes neutral evolution. In neutral evolution, there is a linear relationship between the cumulative number of mutations and the inverse of the allelic frequency (number of sequencing reads that have the mutation over the total number of reads). Williams et al. tested the neutral evolution model against sequencing data from 14 tumor types (904 samples in total) and discovered that 32% of the cases fit this model [5].

Table 1 Main theories to explain cancer evolution

Theory	Hypothesis
Neutral evolution	There is no competition between tumor clones. Neutral evolution is characterized by a mutational load that is proportional to the proliferation and mutation rates of the tumor.
Clonal evolution	Cancer cells acquire mutations over time, some of which provide a gain of fitness. Cells that acquire mutations that increase their fitness will become the dominating clone within the tumor. This competition occurs throughout the lifetime of a tumor, resulting in either linear or branched evolution patterns.
Cancer stem cells (CSCs)	CSCs are proposed to be the only cancer cells with unlimited self-renewal capabilities. CSCs give rise to the various clones found within the tumor.

Solid evidence suggests that tumor heterogeneity plays a major role in resistance to targeted therapies. In this chapter, we will describe the heterogeneity of hepatocellular carcinoma (HCC) in detail and the role it may play in targeted drug resistance. Furthermore, we will discuss methods of detecting and defining heterogeneity that could facilitate monitoring treatment resistance.

Spectrum of Heterogeneity in Hepatocellular Carcinoma: Impact on Drug Resistance

As highlighted by the U.S. National Cancer Institute in their 2016 report, the steady increase in liver cancer deaths is a cause for concern [6]. A combination of rising incidence, limited therapeutic options and its co-occurrence with a frequently fatal underlying liver disease (i.e., cirrhosis) explains its high death rate. The combination of transcriptomic and epigenetic data from human liver cancer specimens allows HCC to be classified in different molecular subclasses [7–9]. In addition, gene expression signatures helped identify subgroups of patients with an aggressive clinical behavior and characterize mechanisms of resistance to sorafenib [10]. Translation of these findings in clinical practice could eventually improve patient survival. However, a clear understanding of the extent and impact of molecular heterogeneity is critical to facilitate the translation of this knowledge into changes in decision-making for HCC patients.

With the ever-increasing number of genetic profiles being collected in cancer patients, there is dramatic evidence of heterogeneity at many levels in this disease (Fig. 1). Inter-patient heterogeneity is the genetic variation between tumors of different patients. In HCC, several studies have profiled hundreds of tumors using next generation sequencing [11–13]. An emerging theme from these studies is that HCC is highly heterogeneous, but genetic similarities have emerged. In recent years, much attention has been focused on the molecular classification of HCC and identifying oncogenic driver genes. HCC typically arises in the background of liver damage caused by viral hepatitis, high alcohol consumption, and non-alcoholic fatty liver disease [14]. Indeed, certain etiologies like hepatitis B virus (HBV) coupled with aflatoxin B1 exposure have a direct oncogenic role in the development of HCC, typically through inducing single-nucleotide mutations in tumor suppressor genes like *TP53* and HBV integrations in the *TERT* promoter. Among the mutational hallmarks of HCC are genes involved in regulatory pathways of telomere maintenance, cell-cycle regulators, Wnt/β-catenin, chromatin remodeling, RAS/RAF/MAPK and AKT/mTOR signaling. Frequently, mutated genes from these pathways include the *TERT* promoter (60%), *TP53* (~30%), *CTNNB1* (~30%), *ARID2* (10%), *NFE2L2* (5%), and *TSC1/2* (5%) [15].

Broadly, HCC can be classified in two main molecular groups, the Proliferation and Non-proliferation classes [16]. The Proliferation class accounts for around 50% of HCC patients and is characterized by de-regulation of pathways involved in cell

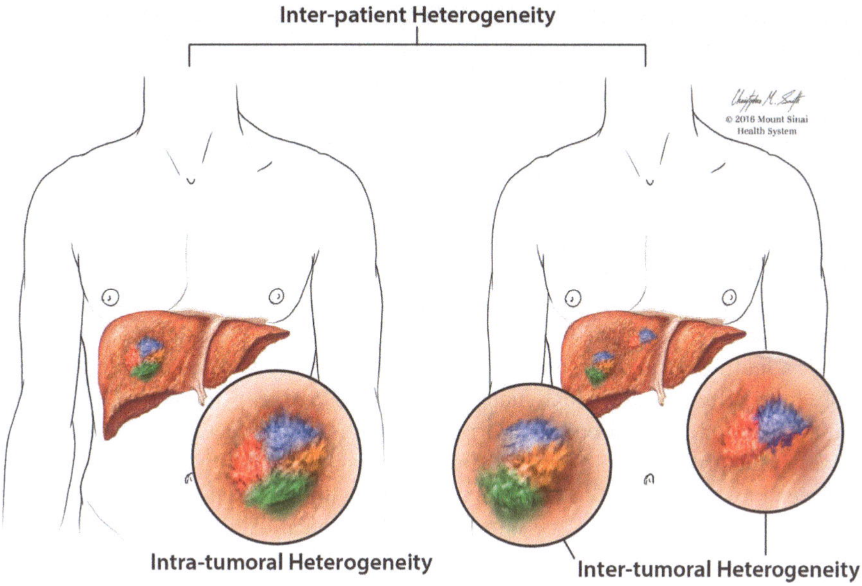

Fig. 1 This figure illustrates the three different forms of heterogeneity that may be observed in HCC. Inter-patient heterogeneity is seen among different HCC patients. Intra-tumoral heterogeneity may be identified within a single tumor that contains different populations of cells harboring distinctive phenotypic and genotypic features, while inter-tumoral heterogeneity is described in patients with multiple nodules that differ from each other

proliferation such as the RAS/MAPK, AKT/MTOR or MET signaling. In addition, this class is enriched in molecular features associated with a progenitor cell phenotype [17]. This class tends to have higher chromosomal instability and clinical features suggestive of aggressive clinical behavior such as high AFP levels, poor cell differentiation, and higher rates of vascular invasion. Oppositely, patients with tumors in the Non-proliferation class tend to have better clinical outcomes. Clinically, this class is characterized by patients with HCV or alcohol-induced liver disease, well-differentiated tumors, and less vascular invasion. The dominating signaling pathway active in the Non-proliferation class is WNT/β-catenin, mainly through *CTNNB1* mutations [15]. In addition to gene expression signatures, mutation signatures have also been described, which provide a more global view on mutational patterns [18]. Epigenetic alterations are also recurrent in HCC, with evidence of promoter methylation-mediated silencing of tumor suppressors (i.e., *RASSF1*, *SOCS1*, p16, and E-cadherin [*CDH1*]), and epigenetic-based activation of the known HCC driver *IGF2* [19–22]. A 36-CpG site methylation signature was shown to correlate with patient outcome, further underscoring the importance of inter-patient molecular heterogeneity [8]. The challenges posed by the diverse nature of HCC evolutionary trajectory is evidenced by the number of phase 3 clinical trial failures in recent years [23]. One of the complications stems from the lack of information on critical drivers of tumor progression and the aforementioned heterogeneous nature of HCC. Other obstacles in previous clinical trials derive from liver toxicity and lack of anti-tumoral potency [24]. Novel trials are being designed in biomarker-based subpopulations of patients with HCC, which is expected to improve the success rate [25].

Despite the insights gained in inter-patient heterogeneity thanks to the HCC molecular classifications, the breadth of intra-patient genetic heterogeneity remains elusive. Understanding the mechanisms driving the numerous oncogenic processes is crucial for effective patient stratification and treatment of advanced disease, including multi-focal HCC. Several studies have addressed the discovery of the underlying genomic landscape of multi-focal HCC [26, 27]. A recent study focused on the characterization of the two distinct processes for the origin of multifocal HCC: a multi-centric disease (in which each tumor originates independently, possibly from different initial malignant clones) versus intrahepatic metastases (where multiple tumors share a common origin and, thus, are expected to share somatic driver events that are remnants of their shared ancestry). Being able to distinguish between multi-centric disease and intra-hepatic metastases could have an impact in patients' outcome and translate into changes in clinical decision-making. By integrating whole-genome, transcriptome sequencing and copy number variation the authors were able to profile and distinguish between the two models of multifocal HCC. More recently, a larger cohort of 47 liver nodules from 23 patients also tried to address the problem of distinguishing between intra-hepatic metastasis and multicentric disease [28]. The frequency of shared mutations between nodules was used to discern whether they developed independently.

The last 10 years have seen the development of only two therapeutic options for advance HCC: sorafenib and regorafenib, both multikinase inhibitors, which targets include B-Raf, VEGFR, and PDGFR-β [29, 30]. There are multiple mechanisms that can lead to resistance upon long-term exposure to sorafenib: addiction switching, compensatory pathways, epithelial-mesenchymal transition (EMT) and cancer stem cells among others [31]. Due to genetic heterogeneity, the prediction of sensitivity and resistance to sorafenib remains a challenging task. Nonetheless, some pathways have shown a particular correlation with sorafenib resistance, like the PI3K/AKT and JAK-STAT pathways. The PI3K/AKT pathway together with MAPK signaling are critically involved in the development of a subset of HCC and are active or up-regulated in approximately 5–10% of HCC tumors [14]. Sorafenib resistant HCCs have been shown to up-regulate *AKT*, p-STAT3, p-JAK1 and p-JAK2 [32]. Conversely, sorafenib-resistant HCCs have lower levels of Src-homology protein tyrosine phosphatases SHP-1 and p-SHP-1 [33]. Other mechanisms like hypoxia and EMT have been shown to also play a direct role in sorafenib resistance [34]. Other chapters in this book explore in more detail these mechanisms. Regional activation of these pathways in heterogeneous tumors could negatively impact the development of predictive biomarkers of tumor resistance to molecular therapies.

Intra-Tumor Heterogeneity in Hepatocellular Carcinoma

Many studies have been conducted using whole exome sequencing of multi-regional samples to study genetic intra-tumoral heterogeneity in human cancer (Table 2) [35–52]. The seminal paper by Gerlinger et al. was one of the first studies to describe branched evolution of tumors using next-generation sequencing data [51]. Multi-regional samples were taken from two patients' primary renal tumors as well as samples from metastatic sites. Somatic mutations classified as ubiquitous, shared, or private were used to infer relationships between each tumor region by clonal ordering. Clonal ordering analysis revealed branched evolution, in which certain branches went on to become metastatic sites. Overall, 63–69% of mutations were not ubiquitously found. In addition to heterogeneity at the level of somatic mutations, variability was found in the ploidy and enrichment of a 110-gene prognostic signature among different biopsies of the same patient. Notably, the primary tumor region of patient 1 that was the closest ancestor to the metastatic site had a similar ploidy and prognostic signature profile as was seen in the metastatic region, whereas the other primary regions were more divergent. This study, added to the others included in Table 2, suggests that the amount of intra-tumor heterogeneity within a tumor has a vast range between individual patients and has the ability to alter gene signature predictions or classification of tumors into genetic subtypes. Additionally, metastatic lesions can diverge from primary tumors at a range of time points (early of late) in tumor progression.

HCC is known to be heterogeneous morphologically. Studies dating back to the 1980s have observed tumor cells of different histologic grades within the same nodule in close to 50% of HCCs [53]. More recently, a study systematically investigated phenotypic heterogeneity in 23 HCCs [43]. Morphologic heterogeneity was defined as the presence of intra-tumor fibrotic septa, nodule in nodule growth, or demarcating architectural growth patterns. In addition, clinically relevant immunohistochemical markers such as CK7/CK19, epithelial cell adhesion molecule (EpCAM), α-fetoprotein (AFP), glutamine synthetase (GS), and β-catenin were assessed. Morphologic heterogeneity was observed in 87% of HCCs. Immunohistochemical variability was seen in 60% of HCCs. This study also investigated if there was underlying genetic intra-tumor heterogeneity in HCC as opposed to cell plasticity being the driving force of phenotypic diversity. An average of five areas per tumor was sequenced for *CTNNB1* and *TP53* mutations. Twenty-two percent of HCCs had differences in mutation status throughout the tumor. These tumors were associated with morphological and immunohistochemical heterogeneities, which suggests that genetic and phenotypic heterogeneity are correlative [54].

A more comprehensive study analyzed 43 lesions collected from 10 HBV-HCC patients [45], including primary tumors, multi-centric disease, intrahepatic metastasis, bile duct tumor thrombus, and portal vein tumor thrombus. Intra-tumor heterogeneity and differences among a patient's tumor lesions were assessed using whole-genome and whole-exome next generation sequencing. Unique and shared somatic non-synonymous mutations were identified among sampled regions of the

Table 2 Summary of main studies on intra-tumor heterogeneity in human cancer

Tumor type	n (patients)	n (samples)	Cohort description	Type of analysis	Main findings	Potential limitations	Reference
Breast	60	122	41 patients (single sample); 9 patients (34 samples); 8 patients (paired tumor vs adjacent tissue); 12 patients (paired primary vs metastases)	Assessment of CNVs using CGH	Developed heterogeneity score based on percent concordance of copy number between tumor regions. Median heterogeneity score = 17%. Clonality profile suggest metastatic lesions diverged early in tumor evolution	Only assessed CNVs	Torres et al. [35]
	3	6 PDX	2 breast cancer cell lines; 3 PDX; 3 passaged PDX	Single cell barcoding of breast cancer cell lines and PDX. Clonal composition assessed by DNA sequencing of barcodes	In breast cancer cell line xenograft and PDX, clonal composition between primary and metastatic tumors is drastically different. Serially passaged breast cancer cell line xenograft and PDX tumors have less mutations than primary tumors. Clonal growth dynamics was diverse over serial passaging of PDX tumors	Limited sample number. Maximum of 4 passages for the serial passaging assessment	Nguyen et al. [36]

	71	181	5 patients (4 samples); 39 patients (3 samples); 27 patients (2 samples)	NanoString nCounter analysis for expression of 141 genes included in clinical gene expression panels	For patients with highly heterogeneous tumors as determined by presence of Ki68 or PR staining, single core biopsies could under or over estimate prognostic risk. 18/71 (25%) patients had divergent risk scores between sections and cores of the same tumor	Multi-regional sampling guided by levels of Ki67 and PR could introduce a bias	Gyanchandani et al. [37]
	2	200	Patient 1 (100 primary tumor cells); Patient 2 (52 primary tumor cells, 48 metastatic tumor cells)	FACS to assess tumor cell ploidy. Single nuclei sequencing to assess copy number variation	Aneuploid, diploid, and pseudodiploid cells were discovered in each tumor using FACS. Metastatic tumor cells copy number profiles are similar to primary cells, suggesting an advanced expansion. Discovery of pseudodiploid cells previously undetectable with other methods	Due to low coverage of single nuclei sequencing, only large structural variants are detected	Navin et al. [38]

(continued)

Table 2 (continued)

Tumor type	n (patients)	n (samples)	Cohort description	Type of analysis	Main findings	Potential limitations	Reference
Colorectal	81	741 CTCs	49 patients (mCRC); 32 patients (nmCRC)	CellSearch for CTC detection. EGFR expression determined using a fluorescein-conjugated antibody	>2 CTCs detected in 24 of 49 patients with mCRC and 7 of 32 patients with nmCRC. Heterogeneity in EGFR expression of CTCs from the same patient was observed	CellSearch method uses only EpCAM, followed by staining for cytokeratin (epithelial marker) and CD45 (leukocyte marker). No quantification of EGFR staining	Gasch et al. [39]
	45	~560	10 patients (early disease); 15 patients (advanced disease); 20 patients (metastatic disease)	SSCP analyses of K-Ras and TP53 point mutations. RFLP analysis of APC. PCR analysis of DCC loss of heterozygosity	High level of heterogeneity in early stage tumors (90% of patients). Majority of patients show same clonal composition across different metastases, suggesting selection of dominant clone early	Assessed mutation status of only 2 genes and 2 structural variants	Losi et al. [40]

Glioblastoma	2	~55	2 patients with EGFR focal amplifications	Single nuclei isolated using flow cytometry. Single nuclei sequencing to assess EGFR copy number and SNVs	EGFR copy number is variable between cells of the same tumor. Multiple SNVs were found in nonoverlapping cell populations	Limited patients and sample number. Focused only on EGFR variation	Francis et al. [41]
	5	672	96–192 cells per patient	SMART-seq single cell mRNA sequencing. MDS to display similarity of expression between cells. Hierarchical clustering and PCA of expression data. Examined distribution of subtype signatures by calculating subtype scores for each cell using classifier gene sets	4 meta-signatures composed of genes that were co-expressed by individual cells were discovered. These signatures were enriched for cell cycle, hypoxia, complement/immune response, and oligodendrocyte function. All tumors included in the study had a mixture of cells that conformed to different subtype classifications		Patel et al. [42]

(continued)

Table 2 (continued)

Tumor type	n (patients)	n (samples)	Cohort description	Type of analysis	Main findings	Potential limitations	Reference
Liver	23	120	Mean 5 regions per patient	IHC for CK7, CK19, CD34, CD44, EpCAM, AFP, β-catenin, and glutamine synthetase. Sanger sequencing of β-catenin and TP53	22% of patients had heterogeneous morphology, IHC staining and molecular TP53 and β-catenin status. 87% had heterogenous findings in at least one of the 3 assessments	Limited number of patients assessed. Mutation status assessed for only 2 genes	Friemel et al. [43]
	1	286	N/A	23 regions were whole exome sequenced and 263 regions were genotyped to determine tumor evolution pattern	Based on SNVs, 20 clones were identified in the tumor that carry unique somatic mutations. Clonal growth rate estimates suggest non-Darwinian evolution of this tumor	Only one tumor assessed	Ling et al. [44]
	10	43	Mean 4 regions per patient (HBV positive). Includes tumor thrombi, intrahepatic metastasis, satellite nodules and multicentric occurrences	Whole exome and genome sequencing. SNVs and CNVs were determined	Ubiquitous mutations ranged from 8 to 90%. Intrahepatic metastasis and tumor thrombus can occur early or late in tumor evolution	Multi-regional sampling of primary tumors was not performed. Limited number of patients assessed	Xue et al. [45]

Lung	12	13	12 patients with rociletinib (EGFR inhibitor) resistance	T790M EGFR mutation checked with next generation sequencing or allele-specific PCR. ctDNA quantified by BEAMING	6 of 13 lost their initial T790M EGFR mutation that is the target of rociletinib. 3 patients developed EGFR amplification. T790M-positive and T790–wild-type clones may coexist in some cancers with acquired resistance to initial EGFR TKIs. EGFR T790M allelic fraction was quantified and tracked over treatment course in plasma samples		Piotrowska et al. [46]
	7	25	Mean of 3.5 regions per patient	Multi-region NGS sequencing. SNVs and CNVs were determined	Median of 30% heterogeneous mutations. 4 tumors had undergone genome doubling events. APOBEC associated C > T and C > G mutations were enriched in sub-clonal mutations	Limited number of patients assessed	De Bruin et al. [47]
	11	48	Mean of 4 regions per patient	Multi-region NGS sequencing. SNVs and CNVs were determined	76% of all mutations were detected in every region of an individual tumor on average. Significant differences were observed in the mutational spectrum of clonal vs. sub-clonal mutations	Limited number of patients assessed	Zhang et al. [48]

(continued)

Table 2 (continued)

Tumor type	n (patients)	n (samples)	Cohort description	Type of analysis	Main findings	Potential limitations	Reference
Ovarian	6	31	Mean of 5 regions per patient	Exome sequencing and targeted amplicon deep sequencing of cfDNA were performed. Gene expression profiling and copy number analysis were assessed	51.5% of mutations were ubiquitously found throughout the tumor. 2 patients had large scale copy number differences between tumor regions. Clonal and subclonal mutations could be detected in cfDNA	Limited analysis of expression data collected	Bashashati et al. [49]
Pancreas	13	~86	10 patients (multiple metastases); 3 patients (primary tumors)	CNVs determined from massive parallel-end sequencing. Tumor evolution estimated using phylogenetic trees	More than half of all rearrangements were found in all metastases and primary tumors of the same patient. There is evidence of ongoing clonal evolution within metastases. Organ specific branches of phylogenetic trees were identified	Lacked multiregional sampling of primary tumors	Campbell et al. [50]

Renal Cell	4	34	Patient 1 (8 primary tumor regions, 4 metastatic tumors); Patient 2 (6 primary tumor regions, 1 metastatic tumor); Patient 3 (9 primary tumor regions); Patient 4 (6 primary tumor regions)	Whole exome sequencing for clonal ordering assessment. SNP array to evaluate CNVs. mRNA expression profiling to assess prognostic gene signatures	69% of somatic mutations showed intra-tumor heterogeneity. Heterogeneity of allelic imbalance was also observed. Expression signatures of good or poor prognosis were detected in different regions of the same tumor	Limited number of patients assessed	Gerlinger et al. [51]
Breast, Ovarian, Lung	6	19	2–5 plasma samples per patient	Whole exome sequencing of cfDNA from plasma serially collected over 1–2 years	Genome wide concordance was observed between tumor and cfDNA mutations. 364 non-synonymous mutations had allelic fractions significantly change over the course of treatment	Limited number of patients assessed	Murtaza et al. [52]

PDX patient derived xenograft, *CTC* circulating tumor cells, *mCRC* metastatic colorectal cancer, *nmCRC* non-metastatic colorectal cancer, *MDS* multidimensional scaling, *CNV* DNA copy number variation, *CGH* comparative genomic hybridization, *FACS* fluorescence activated cell sorting, *SSCP* single-strand conformation polymorphism, *RFLP* restriction fragment length polymorphism, *SNV* single nucleotide variation, *IHC* immunohistochemistry, *BEAMing* beads, emulsion, amplification, and magnetics, *TKI* tyrosine kinase inhibitor, *PCA* principle component analysis, *NGS* next generation sequencing, *cfDNA* cell free DNA same patient. This analysis revealed variable amounts of intra-heterogeneity between patients, with ubiquitous mutations among all regions ranging from 8 to 90%. Similar results were found for copy number variants, with ubiquitous CNVs ranging from 22 to 100%. Phylogenetic trees were constructed to demonstrate the evolutions of each patient's lesions using private, shared and ubiquitous mutations. These trees clearly demonstrate branched evolution in HCC, with some of the patients having longer or shorter trunks (representing amount of time that clonal mutations accumulated) before the lesions become genetically diverse.

These results have several clinical implications. Branched evolution, which has been observed in HCC, is constructed of trunk and branch mutations. Trunk mutations are clonal and found ubiquitously throughout the tumor, whereas branch mutations are sub-clonal and only observed in a portion of the tumor [55]. A majority of targeted therapies available target trunk mutations, which means they should target all cells of the tumor. Due to the branched evolution though, certain cells within the tumor may have developed therapy resistance. A single biopsy may only capture a small portion of genetic aberrations within these sub-clonal populations and, consequently, these resistant clones go undetected. Conversely, sub-clonal mutations may be missed for which targeted therapies exist against, albeit in such a case the drug will only be affective in a portion of the tumor. This is especially interesting in the case of HCC, as a majority of trunk mutations are currently un-druggable [15]. The extent of branched evolution in HCC was directly tested in a study that genotyped 286 core biopsies from a 3 cm HCC [44]. The ubiquitous, shared, and private mutations were assessed and 20 clones were identified. These clones were tested against the null hypothesis of non-Darwinian (neutral) evolution, which would require all of the clones to have the same fitness. In other words, all clones have the same growth rate without competition among them. This can be estimated by comparing the mutation frequencies of each clone to the expected frequency of mutations if all clones proliferated at the same rate. The data suggests that the size distribution of clonal mutations is consistent with the neutral evolution model.

A major clinical implication of intra-tumor heterogeneity is drug resistance [56]. Drug resistant clones have been shown to exist in tumors prior to treatment, so when other cells die by targeted therapies the resistant clones have room to proliferate [57]. At this point the dominant clone in the tumor is composed of the resistant clone and no longer responds to treatment. Additionally, it is believed that drug-resistant clones can evolve throughout therapy and become the predominant clone within a tumor. Only a limited number of studies have been performed to assess this in solid tumors due to the limitations in sampling before and after treatment [58]. One major study was performed on BRAF-mutant melanomas, where multi-regional sampling throughout a treatment time course with BRAF inhibitors was performed [59]. One patient had extensive sampling performed from the primary tumor and nine metastatic sites pre-treatment followed by whole exome sequencing. Branched evolution was observed at all sites as well as unique mutations, suggesting ongoing evolution. In addition, three patients had sequencing performed at advanced disease sites after relapsing while treated with BRAF inhibitors. Variability in resistance mechanisms was discovered among the different sites of the same patients.

A study of glioma evolution during temozolomide therapy revealed that treatment had a great effect on the recurrent tumors genomic architecture, inducing a hyper-mutated phenotype [60]. Directly contradictory to the development of a hyper-mutated phenotype in glioma, ovarian tumors appeared to have very few additional mutations in relapsed tumors treated with chemotherapy. This suggests that chemotherapy was unable to completely eliminate major clones existing in the primary tumor and that resistant sub-clones were pre-existing [49, 61]. No such time course studies have been conducted in HCC to date. HCC is not typically biopsied for diagnosis and biopsies after treatment with TACE or sorafenib are not clinically needed.

Approaches to Evaluate Heterogeneity

There are numerous ways to evaluate intra-tumor heterogeneity. Traditionally, the most prominent method is using multi-regional sampling of tumors, both primary and metastatic, followed by whole exome sequencing to determine the variant allele frequency and copy number alterations for each region. These two measurements are then used to map the evolution of tumors through clonal ordering. Clonal ordering assesses ubiquitous, shared and private mutations from each region and creates phylogenetic trees. Phylogenetic trees visually show the ancestral relationships among the different regions of the tumor. Many tumors have a linear or branched evolution [55]. Linearly evolving tumors have only one tumor region with private mutations, whereas branched tumors have multiple regions. This has now been done in several solid tumor types including renal cell carcinoma, breast cancer, NSCLC and HCC [35, 43, 47, 51].

More recently, in parallel to sequencing technology advances, intra-tumor heterogeneity is beginning to be assessed at the single cell level [62]. This provides an unprecedented degree of resolution to understand tumor genetics. Solid tumors are disaggregated into single cell suspensions and separated into individual wells by various methods such as fluorescence-activated cell sorting (FACS), micro-pipetting, optical tweezers or microfluidic devices. Once separated, whole genome amplification or whole transcriptome amplification is performed followed by library preparation. These libraries can be sequenced with standard next generation technology. One of the first studies to employ these techniques analyzed breast cancer [38]. One hundred cells from two primary breast tumors and one matched metastasis were FACS sorted based on DNA content to determine the ploidy of each cell. Each cell was subjected to massively parallel sequencing to infer copy number. One tumor had three clonal populations with distinct ploidy variability. Clustering between the second primary tumor and metastasis showed clonal aneuploid populations from each site clustering together. This suggests that there was one clonal population that seeded the metastasis. With the knowledge of clonal dynamics within tumors at the single cell level we can begin to identify populations of cells that are drug resistant or seed progressive disease.

Single cell transcriptomics also has the potential to help researchers understand the causes for treatment failure. The profile of 430 cells from 5 primary glioblastomas was recently assessed using single cell RNA-seq [42]. Hierarchical clustering and principal component analysis revealed four meta-signatures composed of genes that were co-expressed. The signatures were functionally enriched for cell cycle, hypoxia, complement/immune response, and oligodendrocyte function. Nine normal oligodendrocytes identified in the study were enriched in the oligodendrocyte function meta-signature. Cells showed a wide range in the expression of each meta-signature. In addition to discovering the four meta-signatures, the authors also tested for enrichment of sub-type classifier genes. All tumors included in the study had a mixture of cells that conformed to different subtype classifications. When applying these findings to transcription profiles from other glioblastomas, tumors that had cells classified into more than one subtype had worse prognosis than homogenous tumors. This study shows that there can be a wide range in transcription programs on an individual cell level within a single tumor, creating the possibility that drug-resistant clones exist even before treatment. One study in HCC has taken a single-cell triple omics approach to understanding intra-tumor heterogeneity [63]. This new sequencing technique simultaneously analyzed copy number variations, mRNA expression and methylation profiles within an individual HCC cell. This technique was applied to 25 HCC cells from one patient. Hierarchical clustering of CNVs, mRNA expression, and CpG methylation all support the conclusion that two distinct subpopulations exist within the sequenced tumor, each with unique genetic alterations from each other.

A pertinent method to assess tumor heterogeneity in HCC is through imaging techniques such as MRI and CT scan since these typically provide sufficient evidence for diagnostics. Factors such as oxygen consumption, necrosis or cellular architecture can be highly variable throughout a single tumor due to differences in environmental pressures as well as genomics [64]. The spatial distribution of phenotypic markers for apoptosis, metabolism, hypoxia, and blood flow can be determined through imaging techniques. One advantage of imaging techniques is that is it a non-invasive procedure; secondly, it is quantifiable. Images created from MRI, CT and PET scans are composed of voxels, which are three-dimensional increments representative of the biophysical measurements that were taken by the devices. Readings from entire tumors can be subdivided into thousands of voxels, allowing for a high enough resolution to determine spatial differences. Variation in voxel measurement intensity can be visualized through histograms [65]. Tumors that have a wider distribution of readings are considered to be more heterogeneous. To assess spatial differences, a technique called texture analysis is performed [66]. This uses a two-dimensional histogram to determine how voxel measurements between neighboring segments correlate with each other. Imaging studies in cervical and breast cancers have shown that tumors determined to be more heterogeneous through imaging were significantly more aggressive [67].

A particularly interesting use for imaging is to assess tumor dynamics during a treatment course. Data-driven segmentation methods called parcellation can group voxels together based on similarity [64]. One parcellation method is a binary classifier that groups voxels into either enhancer or non-enhancer groups. Readings collected over time can be compared for how the frequency and distribution of subgroups changes during treatment. This allows for the identification of areas that are responders and non-responders to therapy. One study that included liver cancer cases applied this technique and provided novel insights into pharmacodynamics of anti-angiogenic therapies using the proportions of enhanced voxels within the tumor [68]. Another imaging study in to reveal intra-tumor heterogeneity was a case study of a single HCC, which had areas of both low and high fludeoxy-glucose (18F-FDG) uptake as determined by MRI scans. These areas of low and high 18F-FDG uptake corresponded with low and high-grade areas by histopathology, respectively [69]. A disadvantage of this technique is that the thickness of slices read from MRI machines is much larger than those used for histopathology. Very few studies have been done correlating imaging data to multi-regional genomic findings. This is a great area of interest and prospective studies would provide valuable information about how these methods correspond and reflect the underlying biology of tumorigenesis.

Another tool that could be especially beneficial for assessing heterogeneity and the presence of drug-resistant sub-clones in HCC is liquid biopsy. Liquid biopsy assesses components released by tumor cells into the bloodstream such as DNA/RNA or circulating tumor cells [70]. Since HCC typically does not require a tumor biopsy for a confident diagnosis, a non-invasive test provided by liquid biopsy is a safe and effective way to study genetic aberrations of the tumor. Several studies have been done in HCC using liquid biopsies. A recent study profiled the length of circulating tumor DNA (ctDNA) in 90 HCC patients, 100 chronic hepatitis B patients and 32 healthy controls [71]. HCC has known recurrent copy number aberrations (CNAs) on chromosomes 1 and 8. CNAs in tumor DNA were used as a marker to determine the proportion of tumor DNA present in the sample. The size of fragments predicted to be tumor from the CNAs was compared to the remaining DNA fragments in the sample. The authors concluded that ctDNA was shorter than non-tumor-derived DNA. An interesting anecdotal finding from this study was the discovery of circulating DNA with tumor-like CNAs in two chronic hepatitis B patients who later went on to develop HCC. Another study isolated cell free DNA (cfDNA) from a West African cohort of 348 controls, 98 cirrhotic, and 186 HCC patients [72]. The authors focused on detecting R249S mutations in TP53, a hot spot mutation associated with aflatoxin exposure. The mutation was detected in 3% of controls, 15% of cirrhotic and 40% of HCC patients. Sequencing of ctDNA can potentially determine genetic profiles of all present tumor clones, including those that are drug resistant. A recent study in lung cancer found several EGFR inhibitor-resistant clones from ctDNA profiling [73].

Several groups have also been able to detect circulating tumor cells (CTCs) in HCC patients [74–76]. HCC CTCs have been isolated using EpCAM and ASGPR antibodies. These methods are suboptimal as these markers are not expressed by all HCC tumors and detection rates are highly variable. A recent report attempted to address this by using a method called Imagestream, which allows for multimarker detection including AFP, glypican-3, EpCAM, cytokeratin and DNA-PK [76]. This method enabled direct visualization of the CTCs, providing additional metrics such as cell size. In a cohort of 69 patients, CTCs were detected in 65% of patients. Cytokeratin was the most commonly detected biomarker and in 28% of patients more than one biomarker was detected. Additionally, the number of CTCs was correlated with tumor size, and authors documented significant phenotypic heterogeneity in the CTCs isolated in some patients. CTCs with stem like characteristics, or cancer stem cells (CSC), have been hypothesized to initiate metastatic growth. One study found how an increased number of CSCs in HCC patients was associated with increased intra- and extra-hepatic recurrence [77].

Conclusion

Heterogeneity in HCC can impact resistance to targeted therapy from different angles. Inter-patient heterogeneity proves that not all tumors activate the same oncogenic signaling pathways and thus not all patients will respond to the same therapies. Patients with metastatic or multi-nodule disease may have both responding and non-responding tumors depending on the inter-tumor heterogeneity present. Finally, HCCs display intra-tumor heterogeneity, suggesting drug resistant clones may pre-exist within the same tumor nodule. Many methods have been developed to assess tumor heterogeneity. Detection of clonal diversity in tumors can provide clinicians with a prediction for the drugs that will have the best response and chances of resistance developing. Imaging can be a first clue as to the spatial differences in metabolism and oxygen consumption. Multi-regional biopsies and single cell sequencing provides high-resolution genomic profiles capturing a greater degree of heterogeneity than the classical single biopsy used in the clinic. While these techniques may not be feasible in standard practice, liquid biopsies have gained in popularity over the last 5 years. Further research is needed to fully understand the impact of tumor heterogeneity on targeted therapy resistance in HCC. Improved technology may make heterogeneity assessment a key element in precision medicine for the future.

Acknowledgement Grants support: AC is funded by a Ruth L. Kirschstein NRSA Institutional Research Training Grant T32 CA078207). IL is supported by a grant from the Swiss National Science Foundation, Foundations Roberto & Gianna Gonella, and Foundation SICPA. AV is supported by the U.S. Department of Defense (CA150272P3), The Tisch Cancer Institute (Cancer Center Grant P30 CA196521), and the American Association for the Study of Liver Diseases Foundation (AASLDF) Alan Hofmann Clinical and Translational Award.

Conflict of Interests None relevant to this manuscript.

References

1. Marusyk A, Polyak K. Tumor heterogeneity: causes and consequences. Biochim Biophys Acta. 2010;1805(1):105–17.
2. Alizadeh AA, Aranda V, Bardelli A, Blanpain C, Bock C, Borowski C, et al. Toward understanding and exploiting tumor heterogeneity. Nat Med. 2015;21(8):846–53.
3. Nowell PC. The clonal evolution of tumor cell populations. Science. 1976;194(4260):23–8.
4. Meacham CE, Morrison SJ. Tumour heterogeneity and cancer cell plasticity. Nature. 2013;501(7467):328–37.
5. Williams MJ, Werner B, Barnes CP, Graham TA, Sottoriva A. Identification of neutral tumor evolution across cancer types. Nat Genet. 2016;48(3):238–44.
6. Ryerson AB, Eheman CR, Altekruse SF, Ward JW, Jemal A, Sherman RL, et al. Annual Report to the Nation on the Status of Cancer, 1975–2012, featuring the increasing incidence of liver cancer. Cancer. 2016;122(9):1312–37.
7. Villanueva A, Hoshida Y, Battiston C, Tovar V, Sia D, Alsinet C, et al. Combining clinical, pathology, and gene expression data to predict recurrence of hepatocellular carcinoma. Gastroenterology. 2011;140(5):1501–12.
8. Villanueva A, Portela A, Sayols S, Battiston C, Hoshida Y, Méndez-González J, et al. DNA methylation-based prognosis and epidrivers in hepatocellular carcinoma. Hepatology. 2015;61(6):1945–56.
9. Goossens N, Sun X, Hoshida Y. Molecular classification of hepatocellular carcinoma: potential therapeutic implications. Hepatic Oncol. 2015;2(4):371–9.
10. Tovar V, Cornella H, Moeini A, Vidal S, Hoshida Y, Sia D, et al. Tumour initiating cells and IGF/FGF signalling contribute to sorafenib resistance in hepatocellular carcinoma. Gut. 2017;66:530–40.
11. Fujimoto A, Furuta M, Totoki Y, Tsunoda T, Kato M, Shiraishi Y, et al. Whole-genome mutational landscape and characterization of noncoding and structural mutations in liver cancer. Nat Genet. 2016;48(5):500–9.
12. Kan Z, Zheng H, Liu X, Li S, Barber TD, Gong Z, et al. Whole-genome sequencing identifies recurrent mutations in hepatocellular carcinoma. Genome Res. 2013;23(9):1422–33.
13. Guichard C, Amaddeo G, Imbeaud S, Ladeiro Y, Pelletier L, Maad IB, et al. Integrated analysis of somatic mutations and focal copy-number changes identifies key genes and pathways in hepatocellular carcinoma. Nat Genet. 2012;44(6):694–8.
14. Zucman-Rossi J, Villanueva A, Nault JC, Llovet JM. Genetic landscape and biomarkers of hepatocellular carcinoma. Gastroenterology. 2015;149(5):1226–39.
15. Schulze K, Nault J-C, Villanueva A. Genetic profiling of hepatocellular carcinoma using next-generation sequencing. J Hepatol. 2016;65(5):1031–42.
16. Pinyol R, Nault JC, Quetglas IM, Zucman-Rossi J, Llovet JM. Molecular profiling of liver tumors: classification and clinical translation for decision making. Semin Liver Dis. 2014;34(4):363–75.
17. Sia D, Villanueva A, Friedman SL, Llovet JM. Liver cancer cell of origin, molecular class, and effects on patient prognosis. Gastroenterology. 2017;152:745–61.
18. Schulze K, Imbeaud S, Letouzé E, Alexandrov LB, Calderaro J, Rebouissou S, et al. Exome sequencing of hepatocellular carcinomas identifies new mutational signatures and potential therapeutic targets. Nat Genet. 2015;47(5):505–11.
19. Schagdarsurengin U, Wilkens L, Steinemann D, Flemming P, Kreipe HH, Pfeifer GP, et al. Frequent epigenetic inactivation of the RASSF1A gene in hepatocellular carcinoma. Oncogene. 2003;22(12):1866-71.
20. Dong Y, Wang A. Aberrant DNA methylation in hepatocellular carcinoma tumor suppression (review). Oncol Lett. 2014;8(3):963–8.
21. Matsuda Y, Ichida T, Matsuzawa J, Sugimura K, Asakura H. p16(INK4) is inactivated by extensive CpG methylation in human hepatocellular carcinoma. Gastroenterology. 1999;116(2):394–400.

22. Martinez-Quetglas I, Pinyol R, Dauch D, Torrecilla S, Tovar V, Moeini A, et al. IGF2 is upregulated by epigenetic mechanisms in hepatocellular carcinomas and is an actionable oncogene product in experimental models. Gastroenterology. 2016;151(6):1192–205.
23. Llovet JM, Hernandez-Gea V. Hepatocellular carcinoma: reasons for phase III failure and novel perspectives on trial design. Clin Cancer Res. 2014;20(8):2072–9.
24. Cheng A-L, Kang Y-K, Lin D-Y, Park J-W, Kudo M, Qin S, et al. Sunitinib versus sorafenib in advanced hepatocellular cancer: results of a randomized phase III trial. J Clin Oncol. 2013;31(32):4067–75.
25. Zhang B, Finn RS. Personalized clinical trials in hepatocellular carcinoma based on biomarker selection. Liver cancer. 2016;5(3):221–32.
26. Miao R, Luo H, Zhou H, Li G, Bu D, Yang X, et al. Identification of prognostic biomarkers in hepatitis B virus-related hepatocellular carcinoma and stratification by integrative multi-omics analysis. J Hepatol. 2014;61(4):840–9.
27. Shi J-Y, Xing Q, Duan M, Wang Z-C, Yang L-X, Zhao Y-J, et al. Inferring the progression of multifocal liver cancer from spatial and temporal genomic heterogeneity. Oncotarget. 2016;7(3):2867–77.
28. Furuta M, Ueno M, Fujimoto A, Hayami S, Yasukawa S, Kojima F, et al. Whole genome sequencing discriminates hepatocellular carcinoma with intrahepatic metastasis from multicentric tumors. J Hepatol. 2017;66(2):363–73.
29. Palmer DH, Llovet JJM, Ricci S, Mazzaferro V, Hilgard P, Gane E, et al. Sorafenib in advanced hepatocellular carcinoma. N Engl J Med. 2008;359(4):378–90.
30. Bruix J, Qin S, Merle P, Granito A, Huang Y-H, Bodoky G, et al. Regorafenib for patients with hepatocellular carcinoma who progressed on sorafenib treatment (RESORCE): a randomised, double-blind, placebo-controlled, phase 3 trial. Lancet. 2017;389(10064):56–66.
31. Zhai B, Sun X-Y. Mechanisms of resistance to sorafenib and the corresponding strategies in hepatocellular carcinoma. World J Hepatol. 2013;5(7):345–52.
32. Zhang W, Sun HC, Wang WQ, Zhang QB, Zhuang PY, Xiong YQ, et al. Sorafenib downregulates expression of HTATIP2 to promote invasiveness and metastasis of orthotopic hepatocellular carcinoma tumors in mice. Gastroenterology. 2012;143(6):1641–49.
33. Tai W-T, Cheng A-L, Shiau C-W, Liu C-Y, Ko C-H, Lin M-W, et al. Dovitinib induces apoptosis and overcomes sorafenib resistance in hepatocellular carcinoma through SHP-1-mediated inhibition of STAT3. Mol Cancer Ther. 2012;11(2):452–63.
34. van Malenstein H, Dekervel J, Verslype C, Van Cutsem E, Windmolders P, Nevens F, et al. Long-term exposure to sorafenib of liver cancer cells induces resistance with epithelial-to-mesenchymal transition, increased invasion and risk of rebound growth. Cancer Lett. 2013;329(1):74–83.
35. Torres L, Ribeiro FR, Pandis N, Andersen JA, Heim S, Teixeira MR. Intratumor genomic heterogeneity in breast cancer with clonal divergence between primary carcinomas and lymph node metastases. Breast Cancer Res Treat. 2007;102(2):143–55.
36. Nguyen LV, Pellacani D, Lefort S, Kannan N, Osako T, Makarem M, et al. Barcoding reveals complex clonal dynamics of de novo transformed human mammary cells. Nature. 2015;528(7581):267–71.
37. Gyanchandani R, Lin Y, Lin H-M, Cooper KL, Normolle DP, Brufsky AM, et al. Intra-tumor heterogeneity affects gene expression profile test prognostic risk stratification in early breast cancer. Clin Cancer Res. 2016;22(21):5362–9.
38. Navin N, Kendall J, Troge J, Andrews P, Rodgers L, Mcindoo J, et al. Tumour evolution inferred by single-cell sequencing. Nature. 2011;472:90–4.
39. Gasch C, Bauernhofer T, Pichler M, Langer-Freitag S, Reeh M, Seifert AM, et al. Heterogeneity of epidermal growth factor receptor status and mutations of KRAS/PIK3CA in circulating tumor cells of patients with colorectal cancer. Clin Chem. 2013;59(1):252–60.
40. Losi L, Baisse B, Bouzourene H, Benhattar J. Evolution of intratumoral genetic heterogeneity during colorectal cancer progression. Carcinogenesis. 2005;26(5):916–22.
41. Francis JM, Zhang C-Z, Maire CL, Jung J, Manzo VE, Adalsteinsson VA, et al. EGFR variant heterogeneity in glioblastoma resolved through single-nucleus sequencing. Cancer Discov. 2014;4(8):956–71.

42. Patel AP, Tirosh I, Trombetta JJ, Shalek AK, Gillespie SM, Wakimoto H, et al. Single-cell RNA-seq highlights intratumoral heterogeneity in primary glioblastoma. Science. 2014;344(6190):1396–401.
43. Friemel J, Rechsteiner M, Frick L, Böhm F, Struckmann K, Egger M, et al. Intratumor heterogeneity in hepatocellular carcinoma. Clin Cancer Res. 2015;21(8):1951–61.
44. Ling S, Hu Z, Yang Z, Yang F, Li Y, Lin P, et al. Extremely high genetic diversity in a single tumor points to prevalence of non-darwinian cell evolution. Proc Natl Acad Sci. 2015;112(47):E6496–505.
45. Xue R, Li R, Guo H, Guo L, Su Z, Ni X, et al. Variable extent of intra-tumor heterogeneity revealed by genomic sequencing of multiple lesions in patients with hepatocellular carcinoma. Gastroenterology. 2016;150(4):998–1008.
46. Piotrowska Z, Niederst MJ, Karlovich CA, Wakelee HA, Neal JW, Mino-Kenudson M, et al. Heterogeneity underlies the emergence of EGFRT790 wild-type clones following treatment of T790M-positive cancers with a third-generation EGFR inhibitor. Cancer Discov. 2015;5(7):713–22.
47. de Bruin EC, McGranahan N, Mitter R, Salm M, Wedge DC, Yates L, et al. Spatial and temporal diversity in genomic instability processes defines lung cancer evolution. Science. 2014;346(6206):251–6.
48. Zhang J, Fujimoto J, Zhang J, Wedge DC, Song X, Zhang J, et al. Intratumor heterogeneity in localized lung adenocarcinomas delineated by multiregion sequencing. Science. 2014;346(6206):256–9.
49. Bashashati A, Ha G, Tone A, Ding J, Prentice LM, Roth A, et al. Distinct evolutionary trajectories of primary high-grade serous ovarian cancers revealed through spatial mutational profiling. J Pathol. 2013;231(1):21–34.
50. Campbell PJ, Yachida S, Mudie LJ, Stephens PJ, Pleasance ED, Stebbings LA, et al. The patterns and dynamics of genomic instability in metastatic pancreatic cancer. Nature. 2010;467(7319):1109–13.
51. Gerlinger M, Rowan AJ, Horswell S, Larkin J, Endesfelder D, Gronroos E, et al. Intratumor heterogeneity and branched evolution revealed by multiregion sequencing. N Engl J Med. 2012;366(10):883–92.
52. Murtaza M, Dawson S-J, Tsui DWY, Gale D, Forshew T, Piskorz AM, et al. Non-invasive analysis of acquired resistance to cancer therapy by sequencing of plasma DNA. Nature. 2013;497(7447):108–12.
53. Kenmochi K, Sugihara S, Kojiro M. Relationship of histologic grade of hepatocellular carcinoma (HCC) to tumor size, and demonstration of tumor cells of multiple different grades in single small HCC. Liver. 1987;7(1):18–26.
54. Nault J-C, Villanueva A, Friemel J, Rechsteiner M, Frick L, Böhm F, et al. Intratumor molecular and phenotypic diversity in hepatocellular carcinoma. Clin Cancer Res. 2015;21(8):1786–8.
55. Swanton C. Cancer evolution: the final frontier of precision medicine? Ann Oncol. 2014;25(3):549–51.
56. Turner NC, Reis-Filho JS. Genetic heterogeneity and cancer drug resistance. Lancet Oncol. 2012;13(4):e178–85.
57. Bhang HC, Ruddy DA, Krishnamurthy Radhakrishna V, Caushi JX, Zhao R, Hims MM, et al. Studying clonal dynamics in response to cancer therapy using high-complexity barcoding. Nat Med. 2015;21(5):440–8.
58. Burrell RA, Swanton C. Tumour heterogeneity and the evolution of polyclonal drug resistance. Mol Oncol. 2014;8(6):1095–111.
59. Shi H, Hugo W, Kong X, Hong A, Koya RC, Moriceau G, et al. Acquired resistance and clonal evolution in melanoma during BRAF inhibitor therapy. Cancer Discov. 2014;4(1):80–93.
60. Johnson BE, Mazor T, Hong C, Barnes M, Aihara K, McLean CY, et al. Mutational analysis reveals the origin and therapy-driven evolution of recurrent glioma. Science. 2014;343(6167):189–93.
61. Castellarin M, Milne K, Zeng T, Tse K, Mayo M, Zhao Y, et al. Clonal evolution of high-grade serous ovarian carcinoma from primary to recurrent disease. J Pathol. 2013;229(4):515–24.

62. Gawad C, Koh W, Quake SR. Single-cell genome sequencing: current state of the science. Nat Rev Genet. 2016;17(3):175–88.
63. Hou Y, Guo H, Cao C, Li X, Hu B, Zhu P, et al. Single-cell triple omics sequencing reveals genetic, epigenetic, and transcriptomic heterogeneity in hepatocellular carcinomas. Cell Res. 2016;26(3):304–19.
64. O'Connor JPB, Rose CJ, Waterton JC, Carano RAD, Parker GJM, Jackson A, et al. Imaging intratumor heterogeneity: role in therapy response, resistance, and clinical outcome. Clin Cancer Res. 2015;21(2):249–57.
65. Alic L, Niessen WJ, Veenland JF. Quantification of heterogeneity as a biomarker in tumor Imaging: a systematic review. PLoS One. 2014;9(10):1–15.
66. Haralick RM, Shanmugam K, Dinstein I. Textural features for image classification. IEEE Trans Syst Man Cybern. 1973;3(6):610–21.
67. Li H, Giger ML, Olopade OI, Lan L. Fractal analysis of mammographic parenchymal patterns in breast cancer risk assessment. Acad Radiol. 2007;14(5):513–21.
68. Messiou C, Orton M, Ang JE, Collins DJ, Morgan VA, Mears D, et al. Advanced solid tumors treated with cediranib: comparison of dynamic contrast-enhanced MR imaging and CT as markers of vascular activity. Radiology. 2012;265(2):426–36.
69. Dong A, Yu H, Wang Y, Dong H, Zuo C. FDG PET/CT and enhanced CT imaging of tumor heterogeneity in hepatocellular carcinoma. Clin Nucl Med. 2014;39(9):808–10.
70. Labgaa I, Villanueva A. Liquid biopsy in liver cancer. Discov Med. 2015;19(105):263–73.
71. Jiang P, Chan CWM, Chan KCA, Cheng SH, Wong J, Wong VW-S, et al. Lengthening and shortening of plasma DNA in hepatocellular carcinoma patients. Proc Natl Acad Sci. 2015;112(11):E1317–25.
72. Kirk GD, Lesi OA, Mendy M, Szymañska K, Whittle H, Goedert JJ, et al. 249ser TP53 mutation in plasma DNA, hepatitis B viral infection, and risk of hepatocellular carcinoma. Oncogene. 2005;24(38):5858–67.
73. Chabon JJ, Simmons AD, Lovejoy AF, Esfahani MS, Newman AM, Haringsma HJ, et al. Circulating tumour DNA profiling reveals heterogeneity of EGFR inhibitor resistance mechanisms in lung cancer patients. Nat Commun. 2016;7:11815.
74. Guo W, Yang X-R, Sun Y-F, Shen M-N, Ma X-L, Wu J, et al. Clinical significance of EpCAM mRNA-positive circulating tumor cells in hepatocellular carcinoma by an optimized negative enrichment and qRT-PCR-based platform. Clin Cancer Res. 2014;20(18):4794–805.
75. Sun Y-F, Xu Y, Yang X-R, Guo W, Zhang X, Qiu S-J, et al. Circulating stem cell-like epithelial cell adhesion molecule-positive tumor cells indicate poor prognosis of hepatocellular carcinoma after curative resection. Hepatology. 2013;57(4):1458–68.
76. Ogle LF, Orr JG, Willoughby CE, Hutton C, McPherson S, Plummer R, et al. Imagestream detection and characterisation of circulating tumour cells – a liquid biopsy for hepatocellular carcinoma? J Hepatol. 2016;65(2):305–13.
77. Fan ST, Yang ZF, Ho DWY, Ng MNP, WC Y, Wong J. Prediction of posthepatectomy recurrence of hepatocellular carcinoma by circulating cancer stem cells: a prospective study. Ann Surg. 2011;254(4):569–76.

Modulating Immune Responses to Overcome Resistance in Hepatocellular Carcinoma

Delia D'Avola and Bruno Sangro

Abstract Hepatocarcinogenesis and tumor growth may result in the deregulation of antigen expression in liver cells that can be recognized by the immune system. The immune system plays a major role in controlling tumor progression, and tumor growth depends on the development of escape mechanisms from immunological surveillance. Several clinical evidences suggest that in patients with liver cancer a strong immune response is associated to better prognosis. In the last 20 years, different strategies aimed to enhance the immune response against liver cancer have been tested in the setting of clinical trials with encouraging results. These included the use of cytokines aimed at enhancing the T-cell response, active immunization using peptide or DC platforms, the injection of genetically modified viruses and more recently, the administration of antibodies that interact with immune checkpoint molecules that stimulate the T cell response by suppressing the activity of T regulatory cells or by preventing T cell exhaustion. The combination of immunotherapeutic agents with antiangiogenic drugs may plausibly achieve a stronger antitumoral activity compared to single agents. Ongoing studies will shortly address the safety and the efficacy of such strategies.

Keywords Immunotherapy • Checkpoints inhibitors • Therapeutic vaccines • Oncolytic viruses • Adoptive cell therapy

D. D'Avola
Division of Liver Diseases, Liver Cancer Program, Department of Medicine, Tisch Cancer Institute, Icahn School of Medicine at Mount Sinai, New York, NY, USA

Liver Unit, Clínica Universidad de Navarra and IDISNA, Pamplona, Spain

Centro de Investigación Biomédica en Red de Enfermedades Hepáticas y Digestivas (CIBEREHD), Pamplona, Spain

B. Sangro (✉)
Liver Unit, Clínica Universidad de Navarra and IDISNA, Pamplona, Spain

Centro de Investigación Biomédica en Red de Enfermedades Hepáticas y Digestivas (CIBEREHD), Pamplona, Spain
e-mail: bsangro@unav.es

A. Villanueva (ed.), *Resistance to Molecular Therapies for Hepatocellular Carcinoma*, Resistance to Targeted Anti-Cancer Therapeutics,
DOI 10.1007/978-3-319-56197-4_2

Abbreviations

AFP	Alpha-fetoprotein
APC	Antigen presenting cells
BSC	Best supportive care
CIK	Cytokine-induced killer
CTCAE	Common terminology criteria for adverse events
CTLA-4	Cytotoxic T-lymphocyte antigen 4
DC	Dendritic cells
GPC-3	Glypican-3
HCC	Hepatocellular carcinoma
HSC	Hepatic stellate cells
IFN	Interferon
IL	Interleukin
iNK	Invariant natural killer cells
KC	Küpffer cells
LAG-3	Lymphocyte activation gene-3
LSEC	Liver sinusoidal endothelial cells
MAGE-A	Melanoma antigen gene-A
MDSC	Myeloid derived suppressor cells
NK	Natural killer
PD-1	Program death receptor 1
PDL-1	Program death receptor ligand 1
PEI	Percutaneous ethanol injection
PFS	Progression free survival
PMBC	Peripheral mononuclear blood cells
RFA	Radiofrequency ablation
SSX-2	Synovial sarcoma X breakpoint 2
TAA	Tumor associated antigens
TACE	Transarterial chemoembolization
TAM	Tumor associated macrophages
TERT	Telomerase reverse transcriptase
TIM-3	T-cell immunoglobulin and mucin-domain containing-3 (TIM-3)
TNF-Alpha	Tumor necrosis factor alpha
T-reg	Regulatory T cells
VEGFR	Vascular endothelial growth factor receptor

Immunological Landscape of the Liver

One of the most significant achievements in the field of oncology in the last few years is the development of therapeutic strategies aimed to enhance the immune system's ability to fight against cancer cells. The role played by the immune system in cancer progression has been known from many years. However, agents that potentiate the immune response against cancer cells have only recently been shown to be successful, granting their approval by regulatory agencies for the treatment of specific types of cancer, including melanoma, lung and kidney cancers. Although we have a less profound understanding of the role that the immune system plays in controlling the development and progression of liver cancer, this major breakthrough is likely to have a remarkable impact on systemic therapies across tumor types.

The immunological landscape of the liver makes this organ atypical among all other organs of the human body. The liver is regarded as a tolerogenic organ, perhaps due to its function and anatomic structure that results in a continuous exposure to countless antigens transported from the gut through the portal circulation. Many resident liver cells contribute to this unique property, including Kupffer cells, liver sinusoidal endothelial cells, hepatic stellate cells and hepatocytes, as well as the different types of immune cells present in the liver, such as dendritic cells, natural killer cells, and B and T lymphocytes. The interplay of these various cell types is essential to maintain the hepatic tolerogenic state. Although Küpffer cells, dendritic cells and liver sinusoidal endothelial cells are the major antigen presenting cells (APC), hepatocytes may also directly present antigens to T lymphocytes that infiltrate the liver, especially during infection.

Liver sinusoidal endothelial cells express high levels of inhibitory molecules and low levels of costimulatory molecules in order to promote a self-tolerance state. They express high levels of the program death receptor ligand 1 (PD-L1), an inhibitory molecule that binds program death receptor 1 (PD-1) and induces T cell exhaustion. They also express low levels of CD80 and CD86, costimulatory molecules essential for the priming of CD4+ and CD8+ lymphocytes. On the other hand, Küpffer cells located predominantly in the sinusoidal space of the periportal area are in charge of clearing endotoxins and microorganisms delivered from the gut. They are able to release a number of cytokines such as interleukin 10 (IL-10), nitric oxide and tumor necrosis factor alpha (TNF-α) as well as reactive oxygen species. All these molecules contribute to suppress lymphocyte activation, expand Fox-P3+, CD25+ regulatory T cells, and down-regulate receptor-mediated antigen uptake and MHC class II-expression on liver sinusoidal endothelial cells and dendritic cells. Finally, liver dendritic cells are less efficient in inducing T-cell activation compared to dendritic cells in other organs. While this tolerogenic state is essential to prevent the autoimmune damage of the liver under physiological conditions, in the presence of liver cancer it may contribute to a weak immunological response against tumor cells [1].

Immunological Environment in Liver Cancer

Hepatocellular carcinoma (HCC) is the most frequent primary liver cancer, and develops in most cases in the setting of chronic liver diseases, particularly liver cirrhosis. Regardless of its etiology, cirrhosis is characterized by a chronic inflammatory condition with an immunotolerant status. In this background of chronic inflammation, persistent proliferative stimuli leads to progression from a non-transformed cell to a dysplastic cell and, eventually, to a fully developed cancer cell. The process usually takes many years and is characterized by the accumulation of different mutations, some of them passengers and other drivers, which confer a growth advantage to the neoplastic cells. The genetic and epigenetic changes fundamental to this process may result in expression of antigens in liver cells that can be recognized by the immune system. These tumor-associated antigens (TAA) include oncofetal proteins such as alpha-fetoprotein (AFP), Glypican-3 (GPC3) [2], cancer-testis antigens such as synovial sarcoma X breakpoint 2 (SSX-2) [3], catalytic enzyme telomerase reverse transcriptase (TERT), cyclophilin B40 [4], melanoma antigen gene-A (MAGE-A)(3), and NY-ESO-1 [5]. Alternatively, TAA can derive from altered proteins resulting from both driver and passenger somatic mutations. HCC cells may present these TAA to the immune system in the context of MHC class I or II molecules [6, 7].

Tumor progression depends on the development of escape mechanisms from immunological surveillance. Several pieces of evidence suggest a high immunogenicity of HCC. First, HCC shows a high frequency of spontaneous regressions some of which have been related to immune rejection [8]. Second, anti-TAA CD8+ cells are carried in the bloodstream of approximately half of the patients with HCC [9], and the intensity of these responses are associated with better prognosis. Third, HCCs are commonly infiltrated by lymphocytes and the density of this immune infiltrate is positively associated to a lower recurrence rate after surgical resection or liver transplantation [10, 11]. Cumulative evidence suggests that cancer progression is related to the exhaustion of the immune response within a powerful immunosuppressive intra-tumoral environment. HCC nodules are frequently infiltrated by immunosuppressive cells such as regulatory T cells [11, 12], myeloid derived suppressor cells, natural killer cells [13, 14] and tumor associated macrophages [15, 16]. In addition, the cytokine milieu in the tumor microenvironment may foster cross-talk among these cells, further contributing to the immunosuppressive status. A gene signature involving down-regulation of pro-inflammatory cytokines such as TNF-α, interferon gamma (IFN-γ) and IL-1, and up-regulation of anti-inflammatory cytokines such as IL-4, IL-5, IL-8, and IL-10, predicts the occurrence of metastasis in HCC [17]. Moreover, liver cancer cells may express low levels of costimulatory molecules such as CD80 and CD86, and MHC class I molecules [18, 19].

Immune checkpoints provide the fine-tuning of the immune response. Their essential role in the evasion from immunosurveillance has been key to the development of effective therapies. Most of them are co-inhibitor molecules that prevent over-activation of T-cells in order to reduce tissue damage during the inflammatory response. De-regulation of these molecules has been reported in HCC. PD-L1 is overexpressed in tumor cells and in APCs of the tumor microenvironment such as T-reg, MDSCs and dendritic cells [20, 21]. High expression of PD-L1 has been reported as a predictor of poor prognosis in HCC patients undergoing liver resection [22]. Overexpression of PDL-1 may, in part, be explained by the release of IFN-γ

[23, 24]. In the setting of inflammation, PD-L1 binds PD-1 on reactive T lymphocytes and by blocking T cell receptor (TCR) signaling it inhibits T cell proliferation and cytokine secretion. The resulting condition is known as T cell exhaustion. On the other hand, the binding of PDL-1 to PD-1 expressed on macrophages triggers the release of IL-10 that ultimately suppresses the activation of CD4+ T cells. Similarly, the expression of the checkpoint inhibitor cytotoxic T-lymphocyte-associated antigen 4 (CTLA-4) in tumor cells induces regulatory T cell activation and inhibits cytotoxic T cell activation and proliferation, which contributes to the immunosuppressive environment in liver cancer.

Modulation of the Immunological Response in Patients with Liver Cancer

Ten years of preclinical and clinical research have led to the approval of only one drug for the systemic therapy of liver cancer, the tyrosine kinase inhibitor sorafenib. As consistently demonstrated in clinical trials, patients with advanced HCC treated with sorafenib have a prolonged survival. This beneficial effect occurs in the absence of a relevant rate of objective remissions due to a cytostatic rather than cytotoxic effect of sorafenib. However, HCC patients either have primary resistance or will eventually develop secondary resistance to this drug. In the pivotal SHARP trial, 50% of patients showed radiological progression after 6 months of therapy [25]. Several agents have failed to improve survival following progression or intolerance to Sorafenib including the multi-tyrosine kinase inhibitor brivanib [26], the mammalian target of rapamycin (mTOR) inhibitor everolimus [27], the VEGFR blocking antibody ramucirumab [28], or the MET inhibitor tivantinib [29] among others. Only recently, regorafenib, an oral multikinase inhibitor that blocks the activity of protein kinases involved in angiogenesis, oncogenesis, metastasis, and tumour immunity (RAF, KIT, RET, PDGFR, VEGFR1 and TIE2) has been shown to improve the survival of patients who tolerated sorafenib well but eventually progressed. An increase of almost 3 months in the median overall survival compared to placebo was reported (10.6 months for regorafenib versus 7.8 months for placebo) [30]. This drug, already approved for the treatment of metastatic colorectal cancer and gastrointestinal stromal tumours, is the first drug that is being evaluated by the regulatory agencies for its approval as a second line treatment of HCC.

There are good reasons to pursue the stimulation of the immune response as a potential therapeutic strategy to overcome the resistance of liver cancer to sorafenib. On one hand, immunotherapy is highly tumor specific since its action depends on the uniqueness of the antigen repertoire specificity. On the other, it may provide a long-lasting effect as far as memory cells are able to perpetuate the response to antigens. Finally and most importantly, it offers the chance to adapt to the ever-changing nature of cancer as long as drug resistance is paralleled with the appearance of new TAA.

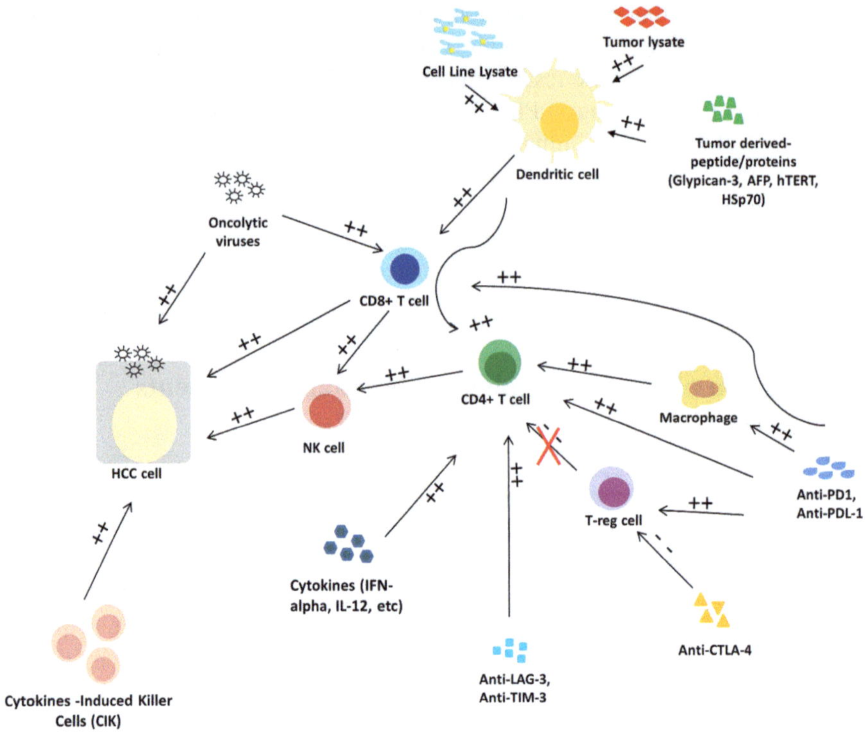

Fig. 1 Different approaches used in clinical trials for immunotherapy of liver cancer. Oncolytic viruses may infect HCC cells and activate the cytolytic immune response mediated by CD8+ and NK cells. Different vaccines containing tumor derived-peptides, cancer cell lines or autologous tumor lysates are administered alone or used for ex vivo stimulation of autologous dendritic cells. Pulsed dendritic cells are then re-administered into the same patient, to enhance the cellular immune response against cancer cells trough the activation of CD8+ and CD4+ cells. Monoclonal antibodies against checkpoints inhibitors may stimulate macrophages, CD8+ and CD4+ cells either directly (PD-1 and PDL-1) or through the inhibition of T-regulatory cells (PD-1, PD-L1, CTLA-4). Antibodies against TIM-3 and LAG-3 stimulate CD4+ lymphocytes that may activate NK cells against tumor cells. Stimulatory cytokines such as IL-12 and IFN-α can be administered directly or using transgenic viruses, in order to potentiate the CD4+ T helper type 1 response and induce NK cell activation. Circulating immune effector cells (lymphocytes T and NK) can be isolated from HCC patients, expanded and activated ex vivo, and reinfused back to the patient to enhance cytokine release, cell lysis or tumor apoptosis

Mechanisms of action and platforms are used to define the different approaches to harness the immune system for therapy purposes in liver cancer. As depicted in Fig. 1, cell therapy aims at supplementing effector cells and consists of the ex vivo modification of autologous cells. This includes tumor-infiltrating or peripheral-blood lymphocytes and CAR or TCR-modified T cells that are later re-administered through different routes. Locoregional therapies including transarterial chemoembolization or radioembolization and percutaneous ablation or intratumoral injection of oncolytic viruses basically attempts to broaden the T cell repertoire by inducing immunogenic tumor cell death. Active immunization using peptide or dendritic cells tries to enhance T cell priming and expansion. Systemic cytokine administration aims to induce T helper type 1 responses and natural killer cell activation. Targeted therapies including sorafenib and potentially new agents may also target the immune system by operating on the tumor microenvironment through their anti-angiogenic and anti-stromagenic actions. Finally, systemic (and eventually intratumoral) delivery of monoclonal antibodies that interact with immune checkpoint molecules achieve an amplification of the T cell response, the avoidance of T cell exhaustion, or the elimination of T regulatory cells. Furthermore, all these strategies can be combined in a wide variety of approaches, which exemplifies the rapidly evolving field of cancer therapy. Only those strategies that have already reached the stage of clinical development in HCC will be discussed hereafter.

Cytokine-Based Strategies

The first clinical trials of immunotherapy in HCC relied on the use of cytokines aimed at enhancing the T helper type 1 response and natural killer cells activation. This included IFN-α, which has immunostimulatory [31], antiproliferative [32] and antiangiogenic properties [33]. In 2000, the subcutaneous administration of IFN-α-2b failed to demonstrate any benefit in terms of tumor growth or survival among patients with advanced HCC [34]. Furthermore, the use of IFN-α as an adjuvant therapy after HCC resection was tested in multiple studies with heterogeneous and inconclusive results [35–37]. The main problem with systemic cytokine administration, from IFN to IL-2 or IL-12, is that the antitumor effect depends on the use of high doses that are poorly tolerated in cirrhotic patients. This issue could be potentially overcome using a sustained local delivery through gene therapy.

IL-12 is a potent inducer of T cell and natural killer cytotoxic responses with a strong antiangiogenic effect. Intratumoral injection of a defective adenovirus encoding IL-12 was able to eradicate HCC tumors in animal models and protect animals against re-challenge [38]. Despite a very short transgene expression in humans using this first generation viral vector, the proof of concept that this therapy could stimulate tumor infiltration by CD4+ and CD8+ cells and produce local objective remissions was set in a phase 1 clinical trial [39]. Taking advantage of the ability of IL-12 to stimulate dendritic cell maturation and activation, intratumoral injection of autologous dendritic cells engineered ex vivo to produce IL-12 and loaded with tumor antigens failed to show convincing antitumor activity [40]. This was partly because the cells were sequestered inside the tumor by the action of IL-8 [41]. Figure 2 summarizes the main cytokine-based strategies used in clinical trials in patients with HCC.

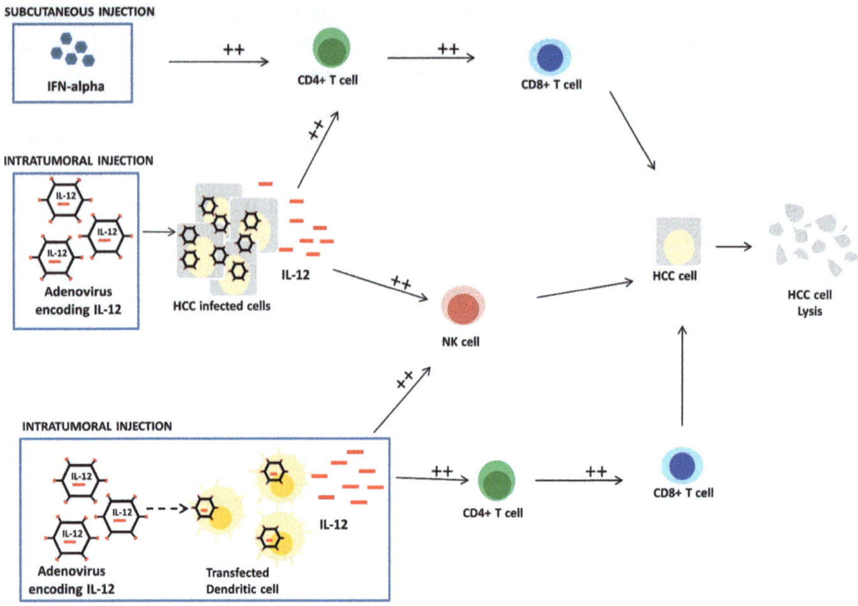

Fig. 2 Cytokine-based strategies. Immunostimulatory cytokines can be administered within the tumor or systemically (IFN-α), either alone or using viral vectors (IL-12). Engineered adenoviruses encoding IL-12 can be injected into tumors. These viruses have a specific tropism for liver cells and infection leads to an increase of local concentration of IL-12; this ultimately enhances the T-helper response and induces activation of NK cells and CD8+ lymphocytes. Alternatively, transgenic viruses can be used for engineering autologous dendritic cells; this can be re-administered in the same patients within the tumor, subcutaneously or intravenously to stimulate the infiltration of CD4+, CD8+ and NK cells

Oncolytic Virotherapy

The use of oncolytic viruses to treat cancer is based on the ability of some recombinant viruses to selectively replicate in tumor cells but not in non-transformed cells, thus self-amplifying their cytolytic effect. Although some wild-type viruses naturally achieve this effect, it is usually obtained by removing viral genes that are essential for viral replication, which function can nevertheless be provided by tumor cells. Building on this concept, the virus can be "armed" by inserting a gene that encodes for a cytokine. Consequently, viral cytopathic activity causes immunogenic cell death, which is complemented by the action of the cytokine. The result is an enhanced immune T cell response against the infected tumor cells (Fig. 3).

Several viruses have been used for the treatment of HCC, including adenovirus and poxvirus [42–45]. JX-594 or Pexavec is a recombinant vaccinia virus that lacks the viral thymidine kinase gene for cancer cell selectivity and produces human granulocyte macrophage colony stimulating factor. Although encouraging radiological tumor remissions were observed in patients with advanced HCC after intratumoral

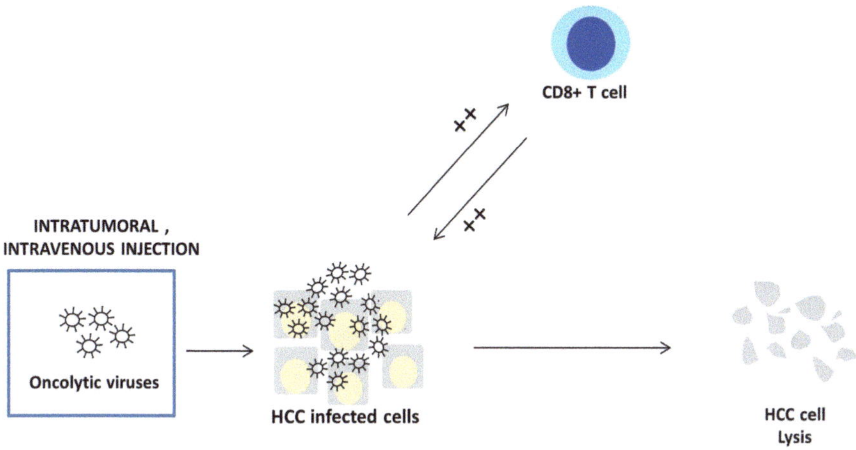

Fig. 3 Oncolytic virotherapy. Specific viruses can be engineered to selectively replicate in tumor cells but not in non-transformed cells. Once within the tumor, the infection can propagate from one cell to another, thus self-amplifying its effect. These viruses may cause cell necrosis by a direct cytopathic effect or through the cellular immune response that recognizes and kills infected cancer cells. Other genes, such as cytokines, can be inserted into the viral genome to potentiate immunogenic cell death

percutaneous injection, a phase 2 clinical trial failed to show a survival benefit in patients previously exposed to sorafenib [46]. Potential downsides include the transient expression of the transgene and the development of an immune response against the viral capsid that prevents multiple administrations. The association of sorafenib and JX-594 was tested in a sequential administration schedule in three patients with advanced liver cancer who experienced tumor progression after two intratumoral injections of JX-594 [47]. All three patients showed marked tumor necrosis suggesting that the combination of the two treatments may elicit a strong antitumoral effect. Based on these observations, a randomized phase 3 clinical trial testing JX-594 plus sorafenib vs sorafenib alone is ongoing (NCT02562755) [48].

Tumor Vaccines

The global aim of therapeutic vaccines is to stimulate a specific cellular immune response against tumor-associated epitopes. Different strategies have been tested in HCC patients, including the use of peptides, proteins, RNA and cell lines as the source of antigens. So far, peptide vaccination has relied on the oncofetal antigens AFP and GPC3 (Fig. 4). The intradermal injection of four different AFP-derived peptides induced specific circulating T cell responses in patients with HCC [49]. Similarly, a vaccination protocol based on GPC3 peptides tested in patients with unresectable HCC was shown to induce peripheral GPC3-specific cytotoxic T

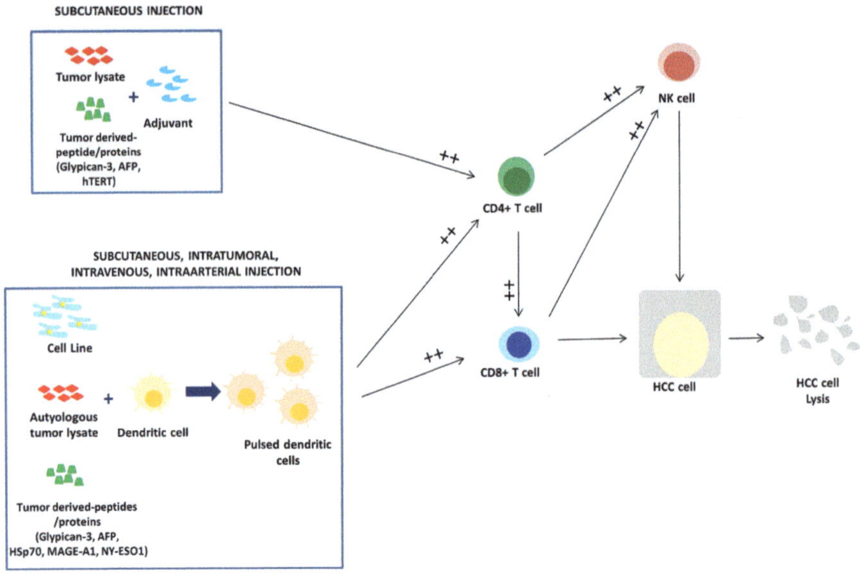

Fig. 4 Therapeutic vaccines. Therapeutic vaccines are prepared using tumor derived-peptides or proteins (Glypican-3, AFP). They are administered subcutaneously and induce T-helper CD4+ activation, which stimulates cellular immune responses. Alternatively, autologous dendritic cells can be pulsed with different antigens including tumor cell line lysates, autologous tumor lysates, tumor-specific proteins or peptides (hTERT, Glypican-3, AFP, HSp70, MAGE-A1, NY-ESO1) and re-administered into the same patient via subcutaneous, intratumoral, intravenous or intrarterial injection. This aims to enhance the cellular immune response directly, by activating CD8+ cells, or indirectly through the stimulation of T helper CD4+ lymphocytes

lymphocytes, and to increase the CD8+ T lymphocyte infiltration in tumor biopsies. Interestingly, the intensity of peripheral GPC3 responses correlated to survival. However, only 1 out of 33 treated patients had an objective tumor response [50]. Based on the observation of increased telomerase activity in HCC cells, a peptide vaccine against human telomerase was tested in advanced HCC patients in combination with low-dose cyclophosphamide to decrease the T-reg function [51]. No objective tumor remissions or specific immune reactivity were observed. Yet, AFP, GPC3 or telomerase are likely not the best candidates for vaccination from an immunological perspective. The identification of new TAA based on the analysis of the mutanome and peptidome of HCC patients is the basis of the HEPAVAC project [52]. The resulting HLA-A2 and HLA-A28 restricted peptides will be administered together with a strong RNA-based adjuvant to patients with HCC effectively treated by resection, ablation or locoregional therapies. A patient-tailored approach in which TAA specific for a given patient are identified and prepared under GMP conditions will be also attempted.

An extensively tested strategy for therapeutic vaccination is the use of autologous dendritic cells pulsed with tumor antigens. Dendritic cells are able to boost both CD4+ and CD8+ lymphocyte responses. An impairment of antigen presentation by

APC [53] and an ineffective tumor antigen processing have been reported [54] in HCC patients. A number of clinical trials have tested the therapeutic efficacy of dendritic cells pulsed both with single or multiple tumor antigens including alpha-fetoprotein, GPC-3, heat shock protein 70, viral hepatitis antigens, tumor cell line lysate or autologous tumor lysate. Strong antigen-specific responses were observed in most cases [55–58] but without significant clinical correlates.

Adoptive Cell Therapy

Tumor infiltrating or circulating immune cells can be isolated from HCC patients, expanded and activated ex vivo with tumor antigens or cytokines, and reinfused back to the patient. In liver cancer, several clinical trials have explored the feasibility and efficacy of such adoptive cell therapy. The infusion of these cytokine-induced killer (CIK) cells has been tested as adjuvant therapy in patients treated with combined transarterial chemoembolization (TACE) and radiofrequency ablation (RFA) with encouraging results in terms of recurrence rate among this study population. However, no validation studies have been performed afterwards [59]. The beneficial effect of the administration of CIK derived from peripheral mononuclear blood cells (PMBC) was also demonstrated in another randomized study where this treatment improved overall and progression free survivals in patients treated with TACE or with best supportive care (BSC) [60]. Regarding patients treated with radical therapies, the results of published studies are heterogeneous. According to the results of a Korean multicenter phase 3 study, the treatment with CIK increases the overall survival and progression free survival (PFS), in patients treated with RFA, surgical resection and percutaneous ethanol injection (PEI) [57]. However, another study showed no benefit [60] in patients treated with surgical resection, but only in those who received TACE or best supportive care.

Checkpoint Inhibitors

The use of monoclonal antibodies targeting checkpoint molecules is without any doubt a milestone in cancer therapy. The interaction between the various ligands and receptors present in several immune cell types and tumors provide the necessary inputs to potentiate or weaken the immune response against TAAs. Upon binding with specific antigens, most T cell receptors induce inhibitory signals including CTLA4, PD-1, Lymphocyte Activation Gene-3 (LAG-3), or T-cell immunoglobulin and mucin-domain containing-3 (TIM-3), while others provide stimulatory signals like OX40 or CD137. Targeting the former with blocking antibodies or favoring the latter with activating antibodies will likely enhance the anti-tumoral immune response. To date, only blocking antibodies reached the end of clinical development and have been approved by regulatory agencies worldwide to treat cancer. CTLA-4

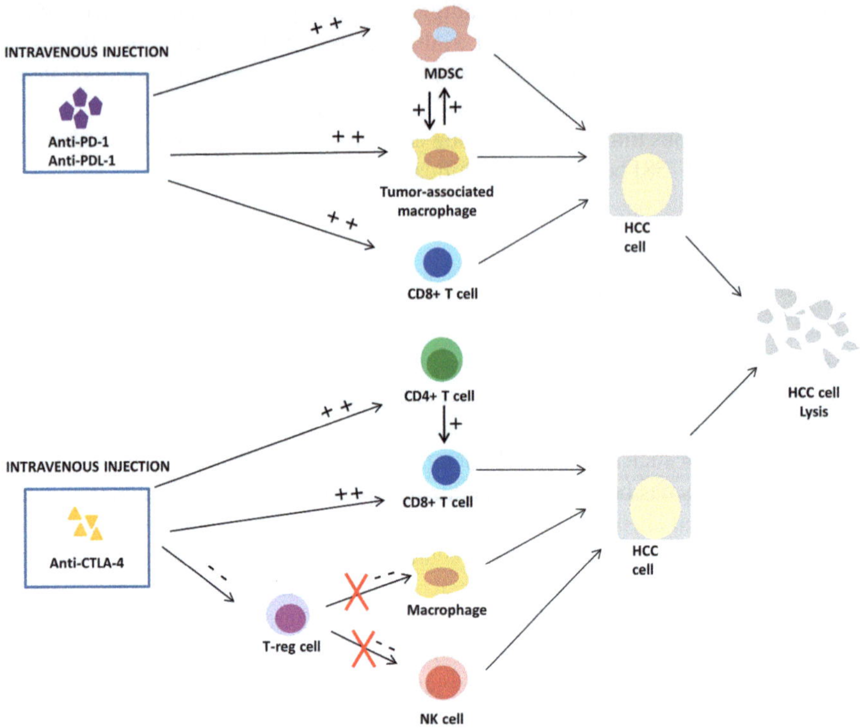

Fig. 5 Immune checkpoint inhibition. Monoclonal antibodies against PD-1 and PD-L1 block these receptors on different cell types, such as MSDC, tumor-associated macrophages and cytotoxic CD8+ lymphocytes. PD-1 and PDL-1 blockage restores the function of cytotoxic lymphocytes and reverts the immunosuppressive tumor environment by modulating the activity of MDSC and tumor-associated macrophages. Antibodies against CTLA-4 restore the costimulatory signals essential for T-cell activity and revert the immunosuppressive tumor microenvironment by inhibiting T-regulatory cells

blocking restores the essential costimulatory signals in T-cells promoting their activity. Moreover, CTLA-4 blockade contributes to revert the immunosuppressive tumor micro-environment by inhibiting the function of regulatory T cells (Fig. 5). Ipilimumab and tremelimumab are blocking antibodies that target CTLA-4 and prolong survival in patients with melanoma [61, 62]. In the very first pilot study of its kind in HCC, tremelimumab showed encouraging signs of efficacy in patients with advanced tumor disease and varying degrees of liver dysfunction due to chronic hepatitis C virus infection (Table 1) [63]. An overall response rate of 18% was observed in a small group of 21 patients with or without prior sorafenib exposure. Additionally, 59% of patients had stable disease that in almost half of the cases lasted for more than 6 months. A median time to progression of 6.5 months provided further evidence of antitumor activity. Moreover, treatment was well tolerated even in the presence of significant liver dysfunction among patients in the Child-Pugh B class. Strikingly, a significant antiviral effect was also observed that

Table 1 Main findings of the clinical trials using immune checkpoint inhibitors in HCC

Agent	Tremelimumab[a]	Nivolumab Phase 1/2 dose escalation trial[b]	Nivolumab Dose-expansion cohort[b]
Target	CTLA-4	PD-1	PD-1
Number of patients	21	48	214
Etiology, n (%)			
Uninfected	0	23 (48)	112 (52)
Hepatitis C	21 (100%)	10 (21)	51 (24)
Hepatitis B	0	15 (31)	51 (24)
Child Pugh class			
A	12 (57.1)	51 (100)	210 (98)
B	9 (42.9)	0	4 (2)
Vascular invasion, n (%)	6 (28.6)	6 (12)	15 (7)
Extrahepatic disease, n (%)	2 (9.5)	38 (79)	161 (75)
Previous Sorafenib, n (%)	5 (23.8)	34 (71)	141 (66)
Patients with grade 3–4 treatment-related adverse events, n (%)	21 events	10 (20)	39 (18)
Best-observed tumor response, n (%)			
Complete response	0	3 (6)	2 (1)
Partial response	3 (18)	4 (8)	33 (15)
Stable disease	10 (59)	24 (50)	111 (52)
Progressive disease	4 (24)	15 (31)	63 (29)
6 months survival rate (%)	64	66	83
1-year survival rate (%)	43	59	71[c]
Median survival (95% CI)	8.2 (4.6–21.3)	14.3 (9.6–18.9)	Not reached

[a]Sangro B et al. J Hepatol 2013 [63]
[b]Sangro B et al. ASCO 2016 [68]
[c]9-month survival rate

was likely not associated with the antitumoral activity. These results prompted further testing of checkpoint inhibitors in HCC.

As mentioned previously, the HCC microenvironment is mainly immunotolerant, which may be driven by the interaction of PD-1 and its ligands PD-L1 and PD-L2. Blocking PD-1 and PD-L1 restores the function of T cells and reverts this immunosuppressive tumor microenvironment by modulating the activity and cytokine production in TAM and MDSC (Fig. 5). In fact, PD-L1 expression in human HCC is inversely correlated with prognosis after tumor resection [21, 22]. Based on these data, the PD-1 blocking antibody nivolumab was recently tested in clinical trials in HCC. Nivolumab prolongs survival of patients with melanoma, non-small-cell lung cancer, renal cancer, and lymphoma [61, 64–66]. This strong activity across tumor types highlights the importance of PD-1-mediated abrogation of immune response in cancer progression. In a phase 1b dose-escalation trial, patients with hepatitis C or B virus infection, and also those uninfected were treated with increasing doses of nivolumab [67]. The dose of 3 mg/kg every 2 weeks was then tested in a large expansion phase 2 that included separate specific cohorts of uninfected patients progressing and naive/intolerant to sorafenib [68]. Altogether, a large population of nearly 250 patients with fairly advanced HCC, most of whom were exposed to sorafenib, was treated. The main findings are summarized in Table 1. Following nivolumab, 15% of patients reached an objective tumor remission, including several complete responses. An additional 50% had stable disease, which was frequently durable. Regarding survival, a 9-month survival rate of 70% was reported in the large expansion cohort while a median overall survival of 14 months, irrespective of prior sorafenib treatment, was reported in the dose-escalation cohort with a longer follow-up. Importantly, these results were obtained with only a 1% rate of severe (CTCAE grade ≥ 3) adverse events. A pivotal phase 3 study comparing nivolumab vs. Sorafenib is currently ongoing [69].

Other checkpoint inhibitors have started clinical development and, following reports of synergistic effects in melanoma, a lot of interest is focused on combination immunotherapy. CTLA-4 plus PD-1 or PD-L1 blockade is being explored in 2 different trials using the combination of ipilimumab plus nivolumab [70] (NCT01658878) or tremelimumab plus durvalumab (NCT02519348) [71], and their results are eagerly awaited. Another phase I study, started in 2013, is currently recruiting patients with advanced solid tumors including HCC to assess the safety and tolerability of a monoclonal antibody against LAG-3 with or without the anti-PD-1 antibody, nivolumab (NCT01968109) [72]. LAG-3 is another inhibitor molecule expressed on the surface of B, T lymphocytes and dendritic cells that inhibits the proliferation and activation of CD4 cells; this contributes to CD8+ T cell exhaustion and dendritic cell inhibition [73]. Moreover, this molecule is able to stimulate the activity of T-reg cells promoting their suppressor phenotype [74]. The association of these two monoclonal antibodies against immune checkpoint inhibitors should provide a stronger immune activation against cancer cell. Results of this study are expected by the end of 2018.

The combination of immuno-oncology agents with antiangiogenic drugs may plausibly achieve a stronger antitumoral activity compared to the single agent alone. Ongoing studies are investigating the safety and efficacy of such strategy. There is little experimental evidence suggesting that sorafenib may modulate the immune microenvironment in HCC. On one hand, in a mouse model of metastatic colon cancer high levels of VEGFA seemed to contribute to T cell exhaustion by increasing the expression on intratumoral CD8+ T cells of co-stimulatory molecules that inhibit the immune response such as PD-1, CTLA-4, LAG-3 and TIM-3 [75]. In this model, the association of a PD-1 inhibitor and an anti-VEGFA antibody indeed resulted in stronger tumor necrosis compared to single agents [75]. On the other hand, studies performed in animal models of HCC showed that the hypoxia resulting from sorafenib treatment may contribute to inhibit the immune response by increasing intratumoral expression of PD-L1 and enhancing the recruitment of regulatory T cells and M2-type macrophages [76]. In this study, the combination of an anti-PD1 antibody and sorafenib was not more effective than sorafenib alone. Another study suggested that sorafenib increases the local recruitment of tumor-associated neutrophils, that ultimately populates the tumor stroma with macrophages and

T-regs, thus promoting an immunosuppressive environment [77]. In this study, depletion of tumor-associated neutrophils combined with sorafenib led to a stronger anti-tumoral activity compared to sorafenib alone. In the clinical setting, the combination of sorafenib and immune checkpoint inhibitors has never been attempted. However, clinical trials testing the combination of oncolytic virotherapy and sorafenib are underway. Undoubtedly, if immuno-oncology agents were able to overcome primary or secondary sorafenib resistance they will establish a new era in HCC therapeutics.

Acknowledgement Delia D'Avola is the recipient of the Grant for Study Expansion from the Spanish Association for the Study of the Liver (Asociación Espanola para el Estudio del Hígado AEEH) and Cancer Research Grant from Nuovo Soldati Foundation. This work was supported by EC FP7 Project Cancer Vaccine development for Hepatocellular Carcinoma – HEPAVAC (Grant Nr. 602893), EC H2020 Project Immunology and Immunotherapy of cancer: strengthening the translational aspect - HepaMUT (Grant Nr. AC16/00165), and project PI16/01845, integrated in Plan Estatal de I+D+I 2013-2016 and co-financed by ISCIII-Subdirección General de Evaluación y Fomento de la investigación and Fondo Europeo de Desarrollo Regional (FEDER).

References

1. Racanelli V, Rehermann B. The liver as an immunological organ. Hepatology. 2006;43(2 Suppl 1):S54–62.
2. Komori H, Nakatsura T, Senju S, Yoshitake Y, Motomura Y, Ikuta Y, et al. Identification of HLA-A2- or HLA-A24-restricted CTL epitopes possibly useful for glypican-3-specific immunotherapy of hepatocellular carcinoma. Clin Cancer Res. 2006;12(9):2689–97.
3. Bricard G, Bouzourene H, Martinet O, Rimoldi D, Halkic N, Gillet M, et al. Naturally acquired MAGE-A10- and SSX-2-specific CD8+ T cell responses in patients with hepatocellular carcinoma. J Immunol. 2005;174(3):1709–16.
4. Mizukoshi E, Nakamoto Y, Arai K, Yamashita T, Sakai A, Sakai Y, et al. Comparative analysis of various tumor-associated antigen-specific t-cell responses in patients with hepatocellular carcinoma. Hepatology. 2011;53(4):1206–16.
5. Korangy F, Ormandy LA, Bleck JS, Klempnauer J, Wilkens L, Manns MP, et al. Spontaneous tumor-specific humoral and cellular immune responses to NY-ESO-1 in hepatocellular carcinoma. Clin Cancer Res. 2004;10(13):4332–41.
6. Makarova-Rusher OV, Medina-Echeverz J, Duffy AG, Greten TF. The yin and yang of evasion and immune activation in HCC. J Hepatol. 2015;62(6):1420–9.
7. Prieto J, Melero I, Sangro B. Immunological landscape and immunotherapy of hepatocellular carcinoma. Nat Rev Gastroenterol Hepatol. 2015;12(12):681–700.
8. Oquinena S, Inarrairaegui M, Vila JJ, Alegre F, Zozaya JM, Sangro B. Spontaneous regression of hepatocellular carcinoma: three case reports and a categorized review of the literature. Dig Dis Sci. 2009;54(5):1147–53.
9. Flecken T, Schmidt N, Hild S, Gostick E, Drognitz O, Zeiser R, et al. Immunodominance and functional alterations of tumor-associated antigen-specific CD8+ T-cell responses in hepatocellular carcinoma. Hepatology. 2014;59(4):1415–26.
10. Wada Y, Nakashima O, Kutami R, Yamamoto O, Kojiro M. Clinicopathological study on hepatocellular carcinoma with lymphocytic infiltration. Hepatology. 1998;27(2):407–14.
11. Unitt E, Marshall A, Gelson W, Rushbrook SM, Davies S, Vowler SL, et al. Tumour lymphocytic infiltrate and recurrence of hepatocellular carcinoma following liver transplantation. J Hepatol. 2006;45(2):246–53.

12. Hoechst B, Ormandy LA, Ballmaier M, Lehner F, Kruger C, Manns MP, et al. A new population of myeloid-derived suppressor cells in hepatocellular carcinoma patients induces CD4(+) CD25(+)Foxp3(+) T cells. Gastroenterology. 2008;135(1):234–43.
13. Kalathil S, Lugade AA, Miller A, Iyer R, Thanavala Y. Higher frequencies of GARP(+) CTLA-4(+)Foxp3(+) T regulatory cells and myeloid-derived suppressor cells in hepatocellular carcinoma patients are associated with impaired T-cell functionality. Cancer Res. 2013;73(8):2435–44.
14. Pedroza-Gonzalez A, Verhoef C, Ijzermans JN, Peppelenbosch MP, Kwekkeboom J, Verheij J, et al. Activated tumor-infiltrating CD4+ regulatory T cells restrain antitumor immunity in patients with primary or metastatic liver cancer. Hepatology. 2013;57(1):183–94.
15. Yeung OW, Lo CM, Ling CC, Qi X, Geng W, Li CX, et al. Alternatively activated (M2) macrophages promote tumour growth and invasiveness in hepatocellular carcinoma. J Hepatol. 2015;62(3):607–16.
16. Ding T, Xu J, Wang F, Shi M, Zhang Y, Li SP, et al. High tumor-infiltrating macrophage density predicts poor prognosis in patients with primary hepatocellular carcinoma after resection. Hum Pathol. 2009;40(3):381–9.
17. Budhu A, Forgues M, Ye QH, Jia HL, He P, Zanetti KA, et al. Prediction of venous metastases, recurrence, and prognosis in hepatocellular carcinoma based on a unique immune response signature of the liver microenvironment. Cancer Cell. 2006;10(2):99–111.
18. Fujiwara K, Higashi T, Nouso K, Nakatsukasa H, Kobayashi Y, Uemura M, et al. Decreased expression of B7 costimulatory molecules and major histocompatibility complex class-I in human hepatocellular carcinoma. J Gastroenterol Hepatol. 2004;19(10):1121–7.
19. Tatsumi T, Takehara T, Katayama K, Mochizuki K, Yamamoto M, Kanto T, et al. Expression of costimulatory molecules B7-1 (CD80) and B7-2 (CD86) on human hepatocellular carcinoma. Hepatology. 1997;25(5):1108–14.
20. Hato T, Goyal L, Greten TF, Duda DG, Zhu AX. Immune checkpoint blockade in hepatocellular carcinoma: current progress and future directions. Hepatology. 2014;60(5):1776–82.
21. Shi F, Shi M, Zeng Z, Qi RZ, Liu ZW, Zhang JY, et al. PD-1 and PD-L1 upregulation promotes CD8(+) T-cell apoptosis and postoperative recurrence in hepatocellular carcinoma patients. Int J Cancer. 2011;128(4):887–96.
22. Gao Q, Wang XY, Qiu SJ, Yamato I, Sho M, Nakajima Y, et al. Overexpression of PD-L1 significantly associates with tumor aggressiveness and postoperative recurrence in human hepatocellular carcinoma. Clin Cancer Res. 2009;15(3):971–9.
23. Zabala M, Lasarte JJ, Perret C, Sola J, Berraondo P, Alfaro M, et al. Induction of immunosuppressive molecules and regulatory T cells counteracts the antitumor effect of interleukin-12-based gene therapy in a transgenic mouse model of liver cancer. J Hepatol. 2007;47(6):807–15.
24. Quezada SA, Peggs KS. Exploiting CTLA-4, PD-1 and PD-L1 to reactivate the host immune response against cancer. Br J Cancer. 2013;108(8):1560–5.
25. Llovet JM, Ricci S, Mazzaferro V, Hilgard P, Gane E, Blanc JF, et al. Sorafenib in advanced hepatocellular carcinoma. N Engl J Med. 2008;359(4):378–90.
26. Llovet JM, Decaens T, Raoul JL, Boucher E, Kudo M, Chang C, et al. Brivanib in patients with advanced hepatocellular carcinoma who were intolerant to sorafenib or for whom sorafenib failed: results from the randomized phase III BRISK-PS study. J Clin Oncol. 2013;31(28):3509–16.
27. Zhu AX, Kudo M, Assenat E, Cattan S, Kang YK, Lim HY, et al. Effect of everolimus on survival in advanced hepatocellular carcinoma after failure of sorafenib: the EVOLVE-1 randomized clinical trial. JAMA. 2014;312(1):57–67.
28. Zhu AX, Park JO, Ryoo BY, Yen CJ, Poon R, Pastorelli D, et al. Ramucirumab versus placebo as second-line treatment in patients with advanced hepatocellular carcinoma following first-line therapy with sorafenib (REACH): a randomised, double-blind, multicentre, phase 3 trial. Lancet Oncol. 2015;16(7):859–70.
29. Santoro A, Rimassa L, Borbath I, Daniele B, Salvagni S, Van Laethem JL, et al. Tivantinib for second-line treatment of advanced hepatocellular carcinoma: a randomised, placebo-controlled phase 2 study. Lancet Oncol. 2013;14(1):55–63.

30. Bruix J, Qin S, Merle P, Granito A, Huang YH, Bodoky G, et al. Regorafenib for patients with hepatocellular carcinoma who progressed on sorafenib treatment (RESORCE): a randomised, double-blind, placebo-controlled, phase 3 trial. Lancet. 2017;389:56–66.
31. Regulatory functions of interferons. Ann N Y Acad Sci. 1980;350:1–637.
32. Dunk AA, Ikeda T, Pignatelli M, Thomas HC. Human lymphoblastoid interferon. In vitro and in vivo studies in hepatocellular carcinoma. J Hepatol. 1986;2(3):419–29.
33. Sidky YA, Borden EC. Inhibition of angiogenesis by interferons: effects on tumor- and lymphocyte-induced vascular responses. Cancer Res. 1987;47(19):5155–61.
34. Llovet JM, Sala M, Castells L, Suarez Y, Vilana R, Bianchi L, et al. Randomized controlled trial of interferon treatment for advanced hepatocellular carcinoma. Hepatology. 2000;31(1):54–8.
35. Chen LT, Chen MF, Li LA, Lee PH, Jeng LB, Lin DY, et al. Long-term results of a randomized, observation-controlled, phase III trial of adjuvant interferon Alfa-2b in hepatocellular carcinoma after curative resection. Ann Surg. 2012;255(1):8–17.
36. Sun HC, Tang ZY, Wang L, Qin LX, Ma ZC, Ye QH, et al. Postoperative interferon alpha treatment postponed recurrence and improved overall survival in patients after curative resection of HBV-related hepatocellular carcinoma: a randomized clinical trial. J Cancer Res Clin Oncol. 2006;132(7):458–65.
37. Lo CM, Liu CL, Chan SC, Lam CM, Poon RT, Ng IO, et al. A randomized, controlled trial of postoperative adjuvant interferon therapy after resection of hepatocellular carcinoma. Ann Surg. 2007;245(6):831–42.
38. Barajas M, Mazzolini G, Genove G, Bilbao R, Narvaiza I, Schmitz V, et al. Gene therapy of orthotopic hepatocellular carcinoma in rats using adenovirus coding for interleukin 12. Hepatology. 2001;33(1):52–61.
39. Sangro B, Mazzolini G, Ruiz J, Herraiz M, Quiroga J, Herrero I, et al. Phase I trial of intratumoral injection of an adenovirus encoding interleukin-12 for advanced digestive tumors. J Clin Oncol. 2004;22(8):1389–97.
40. Mazzolini G, Alfaro C, Sangro B, Feijoo E, Ruiz J, Benito A, et al. Intratumoral injection of dendritic cells engineered to secrete interleukin-12 by recombinant adenovirus in patients with metastatic gastrointestinal carcinomas. J Clin Oncol. 2005;23(5):999–1010.
41. Feijoo E, Alfaro C, Mazzolini G, Serra P, Penuelas I, Arina A, et al. Dendritic cells delivered inside human carcinomas are sequestered by interleukin-8. Int J Cancer. 2005;116(2):275–81.
42. Heo J, Reid T, Ruo L, Breitbach CJ, Rose S, Bloomston M, et al. Randomized dose-finding clinical trial of oncolytic immunotherapeutic vaccinia JX-594 in liver cancer. Nat Med. 2013;19(3):329–36.
43. Breitbach CJ, Moon A, Burke J, Hwang TH, Kirn DH. A phase 2, open-label, randomized study of Pexa-Vec (JX-594) administered by intratumoral injection in patients with unresectable primary hepatocellular carcinoma. Methods Mol Biol. 2015;1317:343–57.
44. Habib N, Salama H, Abd El Latif Abu Median A, Isac Anis I, Abd Al Aziz RA, Sarraf C, et al. Clinical trial of E1B-deleted adenovirus (dl1520) gene therapy for hepatocellular carcinoma. Cancer Gene Ther. 2002;9(3):254–9.
45. Makower D, Rozenblit A, Kaufman H, Edelman M, Lane ME, Zwiebel J, et al. Phase II clinical trial of intralesional administration of the oncolytic adenovirus ONYX-015 in patients with hepatobiliary tumors with correlative p53 studies. Clin Cancer Res. 2003;9(2):693–702.
46. Moehler M, Lee HC, Tak WY, Chao Y, Paik SW, Baron A, et al. Randomized phase iib study of pexa-vec (pexastimogene devacirepvec; jx-594), an oncolytic immunotherapy plus best supportive care (bsc) versus bsc alone in patients with hepatocellular carcinoma (hcc) who failed sorafenib treatment (traverse). ILCA Annual Conference 2015. 2015;O-032:24.
47. Heo J, Breitbach CJ, Moon A, Kim CW, Patt R, Kim MK, et al. Sequential therapy with JX-594, a targeted oncolytic poxvirus, followed by sorafenib in hepatocellular carcinoma: preclinical and clinical demonstration of combination efficacy. Mol Ther. 2011;19(6):1170–9.
48. Hepatocellular Carcinoma Study Comparing Vaccinia Virus Based Immunotherapy Plus Sorafenib vs Sorafenib Alone (PHOCUS) [Internet]. Available from: https://clinicaltrials.gov/ct2/show/NCT02562755.

49. Butterfield LH, Ribas A, Meng WS, Dissette VB, Amarnani S, Vu HT, et al. T-cell responses to HLA-A*0201 immunodominant peptides derived from alpha-fetoprotein in patients with hepatocellular cancer. Clin Cancer Res. 2003;9(16 Pt 1):5902–8.
50. Sawada Y, Yoshikawa T, Nobuoka D, Shirakawa H, Kuronuma T, Motomura Y, et al. Phase I trial of a glypican-3-derived peptide vaccine for advanced hepatocellular carcinoma: immunologic evidence and potential for improving overall survival. Clin Cancer Res. 2012;18(13):3686–96.
51. Greten TF, Forner A, Korangy F, N'Kontchou G, Barget N, Ayuso C, et al. A phase II open label trial evaluating safety and efficacy of a telomerase peptide vaccination in patients with advanced hepatocellular carcinoma. BMC Cancer. 2010;10:209.
52. [Internet]. Available from: http://www.hepavac.eu/.
53. Matsui M, Machida S, Itani-Yohda T, Akatsuka T. Downregulation of the proteasome subunits, transporter, and antigen presentation in hepatocellular carcinoma, and their restoration by interferon-gamma. J Gastroenterol Hepatol. 2002;17(8):897–907.
54. Kurokohchi K, Carrington M, Mann DL, Simonis TB, Alexander-Miller MA, Feinstone SM, et al. Expression of HLA class I molecules and the transporter associated with antigen processing in hepatocellular carcinoma. Hepatology. 1996;23(5):1181–8.
55. Butterfield LH, Ribas A, Dissette VB, Lee Y, Yang JQ, De la Rocha P, et al. A phase I/II trial testing immunization of hepatocellular carcinoma patients with dendritic cells pulsed with four alpha-fetoprotein peptides. Clin Cancer Res. 2006;12(9):2817–25.
56. Lee WC, Wang HC, Hung CF, Huang PF, Lia CR, Chen MF. Vaccination of advanced hepatocellular carcinoma patients with tumor lysate-pulsed dendritic cells: a clinical trial. J Immunother. 2005;28(5):496–504.
57. Lee JH, Lee Y, Lee M, Heo MK, Song JS, Kim KH, et al. A phase I/IIa study of adjuvant immunotherapy with tumour antigen-pulsed dendritic cells in patients with hepatocellular carcinoma. Br J Cancer. 2015;113(12):1666–76.
58. Palmer DH, Midgley RS, Mirza N, Torr EE, Ahmed F, Steele JC, et al. A phase II study of adoptive immunotherapy using dendritic cells pulsed with tumor lysate in patients with hepatocellular carcinoma. Hepatology. 2009;49(1):124–32.
59. Weng DS, Zhou J, Zhou QM, Zhao M, Wang QJ, Huang LX, et al. Minimally invasive treatment combined with cytokine-induced killer cells therapy lower the short-term recurrence rates of hepatocellular carcinomas. J Immunother. 2008;31(1):63–71.
60. Yu X, Zhao H, Liu L, Cao S, Ren B, Zhang N, et al. A randomized phase II study of autologous cytokine-induced killer cells in treatment of hepatocellular carcinoma. J Clin Immunol. 2014;34(2):194–203.
61. Hodi FS, O'Day SJ, McDermott DF, Weber RW, Sosman JA, Haanen JB, et al. Improved survival with ipilimumab in patients with metastatic melanoma. N Engl J Med. 2010;363(8):711–23.
62. Ribas A, Kefford R, Marshall MA, Punt CJ, Haanen JB, Marmol M, et al. Phase III randomized clinical trial comparing tremelimumab with standard-of-care chemotherapy in patients with advanced melanoma. J Clin Oncol. 2013;31(5):616–22.
63. Sangro B, Gomez-Martin C, de la Mata M, Inarrairaegui M, Garralda E, Barrera P, et al. A clinical trial of CTLA-4 blockade with tremelimumab in patients with hepatocellular carcinoma and chronic hepatitis C. J Hepatol. 2013;59(1):81–8.
64. Borghaei H, Paz-Ares L, Horn L, Spigel DR, Steins M, Ready NE, et al. Nivolumab versus docetaxel in advanced nonsquamous non-small-cell lung cancer. N Engl J Med. 2015;373(17):1627–39.
65. Ansell SM, Lesokhin AM, Borrello I, Halwani A, Scott EC, Gutierrez M, et al. PD-1 blockade with nivolumab in relapsed or refractory Hodgkin's lymphoma. N Engl J Med. 2015;372(4):311–9.
66. George S, Motzer RJ, Hammers HJ, Redman BG, Kuzel TM, Tykodi SS, et al. Safety and efficacy of nivolumab in patients with metastatic renal cell carcinoma treated beyond progression: a subgroup analysis of a randomized clinical trial. JAMA Oncol. 2016;2(9):1179–86.
67. El-Khoueiry AB, Melero I, Crocenzi TS, Welling TH, Yau TC, Yeo W, et al. Phase I/II safety and antitumor activity of nivolumab in patients with advanced hepatocellular carcinoma (HCC): CA209-040. ASCO 2015.

68. Sangro B, Melero I, Yau TC, Hsu C, Kudo M, Crocenzi TS, et al. Safety and antitumor activity of nivolumab (nivo) in patients (pts) with advanced hepatocellular carcinoma (HCC): Interim analysis of dose-expansion cohorts from the phase 1/2 CheckMate-040 study. ASCO 2016.
69. Sangro B, Park JM, Dela Cruz CM, Anderson J, Lang L, Neely J, et al. A randomized, multicenter, phase 3 study of nivolumab vs sorafenib as first-line treatment in patients (pts) with advanced hepatocellular carcinoma (HCC): CheckMate-459. ASCO 2016.
70. A Study to Evaluate the Effectiveness, Safety and Tolerability of Nivolumab and the Combination Nivolumab Plus Ipilimumab in Patients With Advanced Liver Cancer [Internet]. Available from: https://clinicaltrials.gov/ct2/show/NCT01658878?term=NCT01658878&rank=1.
71. A Study of MEDI4736 with Tremelimumab, MEDI4736 or Tremelimumab Monotherapy in Unresectable Hepatocellular Carcinoma [Internet]. Available from: https://clinicaltrials.gov/ct2/show/NCT02519348?term=NCT02519348&rank=1.
72. Safety Study of Anti-LAG-3 with and Without Anti-PD-1 in the Treatment of Solid Tumors [Internet]. Available from: https://clinicaltrials.gov/ct2/show/NCT01968109?term=LAG-3&rank=3.
73. Woo SR, Turnis ME, Goldberg MV, Bankoti J, Selby M, Nirschl CJ, et al. Immune inhibitory molecules LAG-3 and PD-1 synergistically regulate T-cell function to promote tumoral immune escape. Cancer Res. 2012;72(4):917–27.
74. Huang CT, Workman CJ, Flies D, Pan X, Marson AL, Zhou G, et al. Role of LAG-3 in regulatory T cells. Immunity. 2004;21(4):503–13.
75. Voron T, Colussi O, Marcheteau E, Pernot S, Nizard M, Pointet AL, et al. VEGF-A modulates expression of inhibitory checkpoints on CD8+ T cells in tumors. J Exp Med. 2015;212(2):139–48.
76. Chen Y, Ramjiawan RR, Reiberger T, Ng MR, Hato T, Huang Y, et al. CXCR4 inhibition in tumor microenvironment facilitates anti-programmed death receptor-1 immunotherapy in sorafenib-treated hepatocellular carcinoma in mice. Hepatology. 2015;61(5):1591–602.
77. Zhou SL, Zhou ZJ, Hu ZQ, Huang XW, Wang Z, Chen EB, et al. Tumor-associated neutrophils recruit macrophages and T-regulatory cells to promote progression of hepatocellular carcinoma and resistance to sorafenib. Gastroenterology. 2016;150(7):1646–58.e17.

Role of Tumor Microenvironment in Hepatocellular Carcinoma Resistance

Leila Akkari and Amaia Lujambio

Abstract Hepatocellular carcinoma (HCC), a malignancy that arises in the context of a damaged liver, is the second leading cause of cancer-related mortality worldwide, in part due to limited effective treatment and the rapid development of resistance. While many studies have focused on the cellular changes that drive resistance to therapy, little attention has been given to the role that liver tumor microenvironment plays in this process. Liver fibrosis, extracellular matrix accumulation, angiogenesis, hypoxia, and inflammation are factors that directly contribute to liver tumorigenesis and can also promote resistance. Understanding the interactions of the components of the liver tumor microenvironment with cancer cells will be critical to design strategies to overcome resistance and improve the therapeutic efficacy of current and future therapies.

Keywords Hepatocellular carcinoma • Extracellular matrix • Fibrosis • Inflammation • Immune cells • Angiogenesis • Resistance • Tumor microenvironment

Abbreviations

APCs	Antigen-presenting cells
BMDMs	Bone marrow-derived macrophages
CAFs	Cancer-associated fibroblasts

L. Akkari
Ludwig Institute for Cancer Research, Lausanne, Switzerland

Department of Oncology, University of Lausanne, Lausanne, Switzerland

A. Lujambio (✉)
Department of Oncological Sciences, Icahn School of Medicine at Mount Sinai, New York, NY, USA

Liver Cancer Program, Division of Liver Diseases, Department of Medicine, Tisch Cancer Institute, Icahn School of Medicine at Mount Sinai,
1470 Madison Avenue 6-111, New York, NY, USA
e-mail: amaia.lujambio@mssm.edu

A. Villanueva (ed.), *Resistance to Molecular Therapies for Hepatocellular Carcinoma*, Resistance to Targeted Anti-Cancer Therapeutics,
DOI 10.1007/978-3-319-56197-4_3

CCl_4	Carbon tetrachloride
CTL	Cytotoxic T lymphocyte
CXCL10	C-X-C motif chemokine ligand 10
CXCR3	C-X-C motif chemokine receptor 3
CXCR4	C-X-C motif chemokine receptor 4
DCs	Dendritic cells
ECM	Extracellular matrix
ECs	Endothelial cells
EMT	Epithelial-to-mesenchymal transition
FGFs	Fibroblast growth factors
HBV	Hepatitis B virus
HCC	Hepatocellular carcinoma
HCV	Hepatitis C virus
HGF	Hepatocyte growth factor
HIF-1	Hypoxia-inducible factor 1
HSCs	Hepatic stellate cells
KCs	Kupffer cells
KIT	Mast/stem cell growth factor receptor
mAb	Monoclonal antibody
M-CSF	Macrophage colony-stimulating factor
MDSCs	Myeloid derived suppressor cells
MMPs	Metalloproteinases
NAFLD	Non-alcoholic fatty liver disease
NASH	Non-alcoholic steatohepatitis
NK	Natural killer
PDACs	Pancreatic ductal adenocarcinomas
PDGFR	Platelet-derived growth factor receptor
PDGFs	Platelet-derived growth factors
PGE2	Prostaglandin E2
PGF	Placental growth factor
RFA	Radiofrequency ablation
ROS	Reactive oxygen species
SDF-1/CXCL12	Stromal-cell-derived factor 1
TACE	Transarterial chemoembolization
TAMs	Tumor-associated macrophages
TGFβ1	Transforming growth factor, beta 1
TIMPs	Tissue inhibitor of metalloproteinases
TLR3	Toll-like receptor 3
TME	Liver tumor microenvironment
TNF	Tumor necrosis factor
T_{REG}	Regulatory T cells
VEGF	Vascular endothelial growth factor
VEGFR	Vascular endothelial growth factor receptor

Introduction

Hepatocellular carcinoma (HCC) is the prototypical example of inflammation-associated cancer, as it frequently develops within the context of an injured liver [1]. Most cases of HCC arise in a cirrhotic liver, which can be triggered by viral hepatitis (caused by hepatitis B virus (HBV) and hepatitis C virus (HCV) infection), excessive alcohol intake, non-alcoholic fatty liver disease (NAFLD) or non-alcoholic steatohepatitis (NASH) [1]. HCC development is a complex multistep process, can take 20–30 years since the initial insult to the liver, and involves different cell types and processes within the liver [2]. Briefly, liver damage induces necrosis of hepatocytes, which in turn leads to reactive oxygen species (ROS) production, cellular DNA damage, and endoplasmic reticulum stress [1]. The hepatic response is accompanied by activation of hepatic stellate cells (HSCs) and macrophages, which produce components of the extracellular matrix (ECM), promoting neoangiogenesis and fibrosis [1]. During chronic injury, an ongoing cycle of cell death, HSC proliferation, inflammation, and fibrosis eventually leads to organ failure through cirrhosis, which is the strongest risk factor for the emergence of HCC [1]. The persistent inflammation and oxidative DNA damage favor the accumulation of mutations and epigenetic aberrations in preneoplastic hepatocytes or liver stem cells [3], supporting the development of dysplastic nodules and their malignant transformation into early HCC.

Multiple cell types (e.g. HSCs, immune cells, endothelial cells) and processes (e.g. fibrosis, inflammation, angiogenesis, hypoxia) participate in heterotypic interactions with the premalignant cells in the chronically inflamed liver to give rise to HCC [4, 5]. The combination of cancer cells, stromal cells, and ECM constitutes the liver tumor microenvironment (TME). The liver TME actively contributes to most key aspects of liver tumorigenesis, including tumor initiation, tumor growth, angiogenesis, metastasis, and immune evasion [6, 7]. Thus, it has been reported that the status of the liver TME can predict tumor recurrence, which affects 70% of patients after resection or local ablation [8]. Furthermore, the expression profiles of the surrounding adjacent non-tumoral tissue correlate with the outcome of patients, being more accurate than the profile of the tumor itself [9]. Accumulating evidence also suggests that the number, type, and localization of tumor infiltrating immune cells have prognostic value in primary tumors, including HCC. While these findings strongly imply that the components of the liver TME contribute to HCC initiation and progression, the body of work reporting the role of TME in therapeutic resistance is much more limited. Nevertheless, several studies suggest that the TME could also play a critical role in resistance to therapy [10, 11]. A fundamental question in liver cancer biology is how the dynamics and function of these non-cancerous, genetically stable subpopulations of stromal cells are modulated and co-opted by developing tumors to favor malignant progression and resistance to therapy.

HCC is one of the most lethal malignancies and there are only five treatments that can extend the life expectancy of HCC patients: surgical resection, liver transplantation, radiofrequency ablation (RFA), transarterial chemoembolization

(TACE), and the multikinase inhibitor sorafenib [12]. Early stage patients are eligible for potentially curative therapies including resection, liver transplantation, or local ablation, which extend survival beyond 60 months. However, recurrence of HCC affects up to 70% of the patients, in part because the remaining TME fosters the growth of de novo or metastatic tumors. This problem is less pronounced in transplanted patients, as liver transplantation removes both the HCC and the liver TME, circumventing the risk of recurrence. However, the procedure carries other challenges and patient survival is also limited [13]. Local tumor progression or recurrence is increased after percutaneous ablation compared to liver resection [14, 15], indicating that the procedure is less effective in eliminating liver tumor cells and/or that radiotherapy may lead to resistance.

Intermediate stage patients can benefit from TACE, which delivers a highly concentrated dose of chemotherapeutic agents (such as doxorubicin, mitomycin, and/or cisplatin) to tumor cells, allowing a better contact between the chemotherapeutic agents and the cancer cells [16, 17]. The standard of care therapy for advanced stage HCC patients is sorafenib [18]. It is believed that the success of sorafenib is due to its dual activity on targeting cancer cells and the liver TME, since sorafenib can inhibit BRAF, but also vascular endothelial growth factor receptor (VEGFR), platelet-derived growth factor receptor (PDGFR) and mast/stem cell growth factor receptor (KIT) [19]. However, these same studies also show that HCCs rapidly become sorafenib-resistant, most probably through a variety of concurring mechanisms that include the liver TME [4].

The contribution of the liver TME to promoting cancer cell proliferation, bypassing apoptosis, inducing EMT of cancer cells, and enhancing chemokines to recruit immune suppressor cells aggregating around the tumor, can also influence drug resistance, making cancer therapy more challenging (Fig. 1). In fact, virtually all HCCs develop resistance to therapy [20]. Studying the liver TME could shed light on how cancer cells turn the effective drug response into failure. Thus, the liver TME could provide cancer with cells signals to restrict apoptosis or develop resistance, and could also affect the drug availability to the tumor mass.

In this chapter, we focus on the mechanisms of resistance to therapy that are mediated by the liver TME and explore how these can be targeted to improve patient response to treatment. We address the effects of different treatment strategies on fibrotic responses, immune activation, angiogenesis, and hypoxia within the TME to understand how they may confer initial resistance or promote subsequent locoregional or distant recurrence. In particular, we provide representative examples of how different types of stromal cells confer resistance to therapeutic intervention in HCC, underscoring the importance of inflammation in regulating progression of this disease and dampening of therapeutic responses. We will review the multifaceted role of stromal and immune cells and their crosstalk in HCC malignancy and recurrence post therapy.

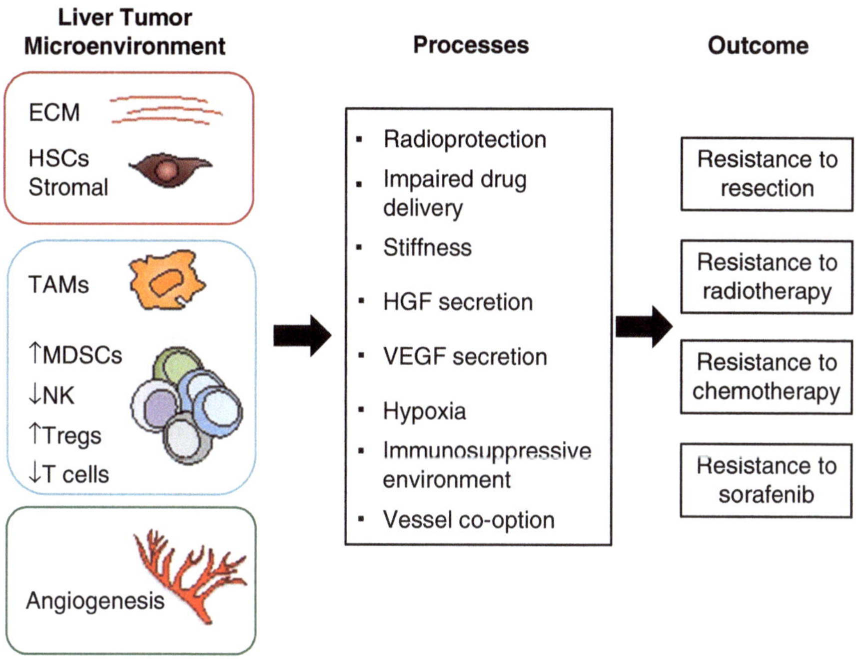

Fig. 1 Simplified view of complex interactions between different elements of the liver tumor microenvironment. *ECM* extracellular matrix, *HSCs* hepatic stellate cells, *TAMs* tumor-associated macrophages, *MDSCs* myeloid derived suppressor cells, *Tregs* regulatory T cells, *HGF* hepatic growth factor, *VEGF* vascular endothelial growth factor

Liver Fibrosis and Hepatic Stellate Cells (HSCs)

Liver fibrosis is characterized by an excessive ECM production and a reduced turnover [21]. In physiological conditions, the ECM is essential to support the architecture of the liver and constantly interacts with the environment, allowing signal transduction and changes in gene expression [22]. Upon liver damage, the liver accumulates collagen, integrins, fibronectin, elastin, laminin, hyaluronan, and proteoglycans, which are secreted primarily by HSCs, but also by inflammatory cells, myofibroblasts, and cancer cells [1]. In advanced stages of liver fibrosis, the liver contains approximately 6 times more ECM than the healthy liver [1]. The excessive ECM promotes tumor angiogenesis, and modulates the activation of immune cells, for example, by impairing the normal maturation of T-helper cells [22, 23]. The reduced ECM turnover is caused by a decreased in the activity of ECM-removing metalloproteinases (MMPs) due to an overexpression of their specific tissue inhibitor of metalloproteinases (TIMPs) [1]. Both MMPs and TIMPs are secreted by HSCs [24] and other stromal cells, such as cancer-associated fibroblasts (CAFs) [25]. Therefore, the imbalance between MMPs and TIMPs leads to a fibrotic microenvironment characterized by increased stiffness that can influence the pathogenesis of liver diseases [26], malignant transformation [27], plays an important role in the ability of tumors to invade and metastasize [28], and can affect the sensitivity of tumor cells to drug treatment. HSCs also secrete platelet-derived growth factors (PDGFs), transforming growth factor, beta 1 (TGFβ1), fibroblast growth factors (FGFs) and vascular endothelial growth factor (VEGF), which can ultimately favor hypoxia [4].

The accumulation of ECM proteins, HSCs, and inflammatory cells can create a physical barrier that isolates the tumor cells from drug delivery. The compression of vessels by solid stress creates two potential barriers to drug delivery [29]. On one hand, the collapse of blood vessels hinders access of systemically administered drugs. This collapse explains why tumors with more ECM might be more resistant to treatment. For instance, pancreatic ductal adenocarcinomas PDAC, chondrosarcomas, and chordomas are rich in ECM and respond poorly to chemotherapy [30–32]. On the other hand, the lack of lymphatic vessel function reduces drainage, leading to an increase in interstitial fluid pressure. As a result, the transport of therapeutics that rely on diffusion, like antibodies and nanoparticles, is significantly reduced [29].

Regarding the role of the ECM on resistance to therapy, malignancies with a pronounced desmoplastic reaction could potentially be inherently radioresistant owing, in part, to integrin-mediated interactions between cancer cells, stromal cells, and the surrounding ECM [33]. Several studies have implicated β1 integrin, a component of the ECM, in tumor survival following radiotherapy [34, 35]. For example, it was proposed that β1 integrin signalling in PDAC can promote stromal-mediated radioprotection [36], and similar strategies could be in place affecting the response of HCC patients to RFA. Cathepsins have also been shown to be crucial regulators of the therapeutic response that leads to TME-mediated therapeutic resistance [37]. This can occur either through intrinsic resistance, whereby cathepsin activity within the TME is sufficient to mediate survival signals, or through adaptive mechanisms, whereby the therapeutic insult triggers a reactive increase in cathepsin activity within the TME.

In HCC, matrix stiffness which is characteristic of inflammation and fibrosis, seems to regulate HCC cell proliferation and chemotherapeutic response [38]. Using an in vitro system of "mechanically tunable" matrix-coated polyacrylamide gels, matrix stiffness was modeled across a pathophysiologically relevant range, corresponding to values encountered in normal and fibrotic livers. Increasing matrix stiffness was found to promote HCC cell proliferation. Most importantly, following treatment with cisplatin, there was a reduction in apoptosis in HCC cells cultured on stiff versus soft supports, proving that matrix stiffness can in fact promote resistance to HCC therapy. The causal role of ECM stiffness in resistance to therapy in HCC is further highlighted in a study where resistance of the HCC cell line Hep3B to sorafenib was mediated by β1 integrin and its downstream effector JNK [39].

Stromal cells can also mediate resistance to molecular therapies by secreting growth factors that can promote aggressive neoplastic cell behavior, stimulate survival responses and prevent apoptosis [4]. For example, in melanomas expressing mutant BRAF that respond to vemurafenib, hepatocyte growth factor (HGF) secretion by stromal cells conferred resistance to vemurafenib-induced cell death [40, 41], illustrating the importance of stroma-derived resistance to chemotherapy, in different organs and different malignancies. In HCC, HSCs can mediate resistance to chemotherapy or sorafenib also through the secretion of HGF. In two independent studies [42, 43], in co-culture experiments of human HCC cell lines and human HSCs, LX2 co-culture significantly induced sorafenib and cisplatin resistance through the secretion of HGF. In fact, exogenous HGF could also induce resistance, by decreasing apoptosis. Taken together, in the search for key driver mutations in HCC, the effect of the ECM and stromal cells should not be underestimated.

Inflammation and Immune Cells

Tumor Associated Macrophages

One of the most prominent stromal cells in the liver TME are the tumor-associated macrophages (TAMs). Macrophages are highly plastic cells, whose activation or "polarization" defines their functions within the TME [44]. In response to inflammation, injury or infection, macrophages are activated to adopt different polarization states [45]: M1 or classically-activated macrophages are generally considered to be critical for tumor cell clearance, while M2 or alternatively-activated macrophages are proposed to have tumor-promoting functions [46, 47]. These polarization states are elicited by Th1 (e.g. IFNγ) and Th2 (e.g. IL-4, IL-13) cytokines, respectively [46, 48]. Macrophage activation can be fine-tuned in response to different tissue microenvironments and to homeostasis perturbations faced by the tissue [46]. The liver resident macrophages, known as Kupffer cells (KCs), are the first line of defense in direct contact with the systemic circulation. However, the hepatic macrophage pool is expanded during liver injury and regeneration through active infiltration of bone marrow-derived macrophages (BMDMs) [49, 50].

In HCC, macrophage numbers are increased and M2 polarization has been associated with invasion and poor patient prognosis [51]. However, M1-like pro-inflammatory macrophages are also found in these tumors, suggesting that in HCC, KCs and/or infiltrating BMDMs can be activated to adopt alternative polarization states. The versatile polarization status of macrophages in HCC could be related to the etiology of these tumors, which typically develop in the context of inflamed, injured livers that share traits with chronic regeneration. High density of macrophages and expression of M-CSF (a key cytokine regulating macrophage biology [52]) in the peritumoral liver tissue, but not in tumor tissue, was in fact associated with a high incidence of intrahepatic metastasis and poor survival after resection [53].

The main mechanism by which TAMs could contribute to resistance to therapy in HCC is through the secretion of inflammatory molecules that affect tumor cells or other components of the liver TME. For example, sorafenib induces host immunosuppression [54–56], and as a consequence, immunomodulation has been proposed as a strategy to stimulate the host stroma in that context. Thus, preliminary studies have shown that TLR3 agonists trigger the activation of multiple immune cells in the HCC environment, including macrophages, and increase the efficacy of sorafenib treatment [57, 58]. In a different study, sorafenib treatment efficiently inhibited tumor growth and lung metastasis, but also increased intratumoral macrophage infiltration. This infiltration was associated with increased expression of the angiogenic factors stromal-cell-derived factor 1 (SDF-1/CXCL12) and VEGF, supporting the hypothesis that TAMs are involved in sorafenib resistance and recurrence post-therapy. In fact, TAM depletion by zoledronic acid or clodronate liposomes, in combination with sorafenib, further reduced tumor growth, lung metastasis, and tumor angiogenesis [59]. Similarly, the direct inhibition of the SDF-1 and C-X-C motif chemokine receptor 4 (CXCR4) pathway using the FDA-approved drug AMD3100 limited the number of infiltrating TAMs in sorafenib-treated tumors and their M2-like protumorigenic phenotype, leading to an increase in overall survival [60].

Noteworthy, contradictory reports have suggested that sorafenib can prime HCC macrophages to elicit a proinflammatory response and enhance cytotoxic NK cell activity [61]. Moreover, a recent study has shown that a subclass of HCCs carrying *VEGFA* amplifications is more sensitive to treatment with sorafenib, possibly via an effect of the drug on macrophage M2 polarization [61]. These results raise the important question of bimodal effects on tumor associated macrophages that could depend on the timing of the response to sorafenib, and in general, to anti-cancer treatments. For instance, in the course of liver regeneration, in a well-described and defined model of liver injury induced by carbon tetrachloride (CCl_4) causing inflammation and fibrosis, macrophage depletion was associated with extensive loss of matrix components during the injury phase. However, depletion post injury, during the recovery phase, limited matrix degradation and perisinusoidal fibrosis [49]. Thus, macrophages can adopt distinct activities with opposed functions during hepatic injury, which can be paralleled to their proinflammatory or immunosuppressive functions in resistance to sorafenib. Altogether, these results highlight the intercellular connection between cancer cells and macrophages in HCC progression. They also shed light into the molecular mechanisms of how tyrosine kinase inhibitors, while eliciting anticancer effects in early onsets on treatment, can modulate the large macrophage pool present in HCC to support therapeutic resistance and disease recurrence.

Myeloid Derived Suppressor Cells

Myeloid derived suppressor cells (MDSCs) are heterogeneous immature myeloid cells comprised by myeloid progenitors and precursors of macrophages, granulocytes, and dendritic cells (DCs) [62]. The main reported function of MDSCs in solid tumors is their ability to suppress specific and unrelated cytotoxic T lymphocyte

(CTL) responses. In acute hepatitis, MDSC can limit immunogenic T cell responses and subsequent tissue injury, and in patients with chronic HCV infection [63, 64], MDSCs favor viral persistence, highlighting their immunosuppressive role in different settings. In mouse models of liver cancer, the timing of MDSC accumulation seems to be highly dependent on the tumor model studied [65]. It has been shown that expansion of the MDSC pool can be induced by secretion of prostaglandin E2 (PGE2) by HSCs in the liver TME. Consequently, blockade of PGE2 inhibited HSC-induced MDSC accumulation and HCC growth [66]. In HCC therapy, an immunostimulatory treatment with agonistic CD137, a member of the tumor necrosis factor (TNF) receptor family, leads to increased efficacy when combined with depletion of MDSCs [67]. Importantly, patients with a low infiltration of MDSCs had a significantly longer overall survival time following TACE [68], or RFA [69]. Thus, in the context of response to hepatocyte cell death induced by therapeutic interventions, it is likely that MDSCs represent promising therapeutic targets to control resistance. However, more extensive research is needed before MDSC targeting approaches can be used in clinical settings to overcome resistance to HCC therapy.

Natural Killer Cells

Natural killer (NK) cells are innate lymphoid immune cells with natural cytotoxicity and regulatory functions. NK cells, together with myeloid cells and more precisely macrophages, form the first line of defense against acute injury and are amongst the first mobilized cells in tumors [6]. NK cells account for a large part of the total innate immune lymphocytes [including NK, NK T-cells (NKT) and $\gamma\delta$T cells], which represent about 50% of the total number of liver lymphocytes in steady state [70]. Following tumor resection, NK cell cytotoxicity is significantly reduced [71] and this correlates with increased metastatic incidence, demonstrating that the anti-tumorigenic functions of NK cells can be disrupted with standard-of-care treatment regimens. While this phenomenon has not been shown yet in HCC, a similar mechanism of dampening NK cell cytolytic functions might occur following HCC resection, and thus, therapies that opt to harness NK population activity following surgery may provide an opportunity to improve HCC therapeutic efficacy at early stages of treatment. Pioneering studies have shown that infiltrating or resident NK cells in HCC patients were defective in cytotoxicity and cytokine secretion compared with NK cells from healthy individuals, and decreased NK cell activity might be associated with HCC invasion and recurrence [72–74]. Moreover, NK cells mediate the therapeutic efficacy of sorafenib in the context of combination therapy using anti-PD-L1 monoclonal antibody (mAb) [75], further emphasizing that reduced NK activity is a mechanism of resistance to HCC therapy.

Regulatory T Cells

Regulatory T cells, or T_{REG} cells, are a subtype of $CD4^{+}FoxP3^{+}$ T cells that play divergent roles during tumorigenesis. The pro-tumorigenic roles of T_{REG} cells include the release of immunosuppressive factors, such as T_H2 cytokines, which disrupt antigen presentation by antigen-presenting cells (APCs) and impair the anti-tumorigenic effects of $CD8^{+}$ cytotoxic T cells and NK cells. Interestingly, the number of T_{REG} cells positively correlates with tumor size in HCC [76] and T_{REG} cells inhibit CD3/CD28 stimulated $CD8^{+}$ T cell proliferation, activation, and production of granzymes and perforin through IL-10 secretion [77]. Both in HCC tumors and in peripheral blood, T_{REG} numbers are increased in HCC patients [78, 79]. Increased T_{REG} cell infiltrates are associated with reduced overall survival in HCC, amongst other tumors [77, 80], and depletion of T_{REG} enhanced anti-tumor immunity in an orthotopic model of HCC increased frequency of tumor-specific $CD8^{+}$ T cells and $CD11c^{+}$ dendritic cells and enhanced the production of IL-12 and IFN-γ within the tumor [81]. Recently, a direct role of C-X-C motif chemokine ligand 10 (CXCL10)/C-X-C motif chemokine receptor 3 (CXCR3) signaling has been reported in the mobilization and recruitment of T_{REG} cells, which is also associated with tumor recurrence following liver transplantation in HCC patients [82]. However, in sorafenib-treated patients, the numbers of tumor infiltrating T_{REG} are decreased [54], potentially through sorafenib-mediated inhibition of the TGFβ1 signaling pathway. Thus, it appears that the role and mobilization of these cells is context and therapy dependent, and whether a T_{REG}-deprived liver TME could benefit response to therapeutic intervention in HCC patients remains to be clarified.

Effector T Cells

T lymphocytes, including CD4+ T helper cells and CD8+ cytotoxic T cells, are key actors in the clearance of tumor cells. Thus, their presence or recruitment in solid tumors correlates with a favorable prognosis in many cancers, including HCC. Peripheral and tissue infiltrating CD4+ cytotoxic T cells are found in HCC patients only at early stage disease, but their numbers and activities are progressively decreased due to increased numbers of T_{REG} cells. The reduced presence of CD4+ cytotoxic T cells represents an independent predictor for survival and recurrence in HCC patients [83, 84]. Following liver transplantation therapy in HCC patients, the monitoring of CD4+ T cells can predict the risk of recurrence [85]. The impact of sorafenib on CD4 T cell responses is controversial and appears to be dose dependent and linked to modulation of the T_{REG} compartment [86]. In HCC, the density of intra-tumoral total (CD3+) and cytotoxic (CD8+) T lymphocytes after curative resection is associated with relapse-free survival in patients [87]. The regulation of $CD8^{+}$ T cell function and antitumor immunity is dependent on co-stimulatory molecules found on APCs, such as DCs or macrophages. These molecules can be harnessed to induce CD8+ cytotoxicity, as reported in melanoma or lung cancers [88]. It has been shown that the expression of PD-1, a co-inhibitory regulator of effector T cells, on the surface of DCs leads to suppression of IL-2 and IFNγ secretion by CD8 T cells and inhibits CD8 T cell proliferation in a mouse model of HCC [89]. Moreover, anti-PD-1 immunotherapy can be of interest to complement sorafenib therapy in treating HCC patients, in order to target sorafenib-resistant tumors that present increased CD8 T cell numbers with high immunosuppressive expression of PD-1 [90].

Angiogenesis and Hypoxia

HCC is a highly vascularized tumor and angiogenesis plays an important role in tumor growth [4]. During the growth of tumor tissues, endothelial cells (ECs) are activated and become proliferative to form new vessels within the stroma, to provide nutrients and oxygen for tumors [91]. Blood vessels in tumors are frequently dilated and tortuous and, compared with normal tissues, have aberrant branching patterns [92]. These abnormalities make tumor vessels leaky, although their permeability varies both within and among tumors [93]. Furthermore, the compression of blood vessels by cancer cells, stromal cells, and ECM [94], increases resistance to blood flow and impair blood supply to the tumor. As a result, there is reduction in delivery of nutrient metabolites and in the clearance of breakdown products of metabolism, leading to hypoxic and acidic regions in tumors. Delivery of anticancer drugs is similarly compromised [95] and tumor responsiveness to chemotherapy is influenced both directly and indirectly by the abnormal vasculature. As an example, in HCC, CD105+ ECs present features of increased angiogenesis activity with higher resistance to chemotherapeutic agents and to angiogenesis inhibitors [96], suggesting that ECs are also involved in resistance to therapy.

An intriguing theory that could explain intrinsic resistance to anti-angiogenic drugs, such as sorafenib, is "vessel co-option", which is the ability of tumors to hijack the existing vasculature in organs such as the lungs or liver, limiting the need for sprouting angiogenesis [97]. In an in vivo model of HCC, sorafenib initially inhibited angiogenesis and stabilized tumor growth [98]. However, no angiogenic 'rebound' effect was observed during development of resistance unless therapy was stopped. Instead, resistant tumors became more locally invasive, which facilitated extensive incorporation of liver parenchyma and the co-option of liver-associated vessels. This study could have important implications including the potential therapeutic benefits of targeting vessel co-option in conjunction with VEGFR signaling.

Angiogenesis is promoted by VEGF, the most critical proangiogenic factor that is strongly secreted after chronic liver injury and also promotes fibrogenesis [4]. VEGF, the main target of the multikinases inhibitor sorafenib [19], can function as a cytokine that directly affects HSCs, KCs, and hepatocytes [99], and mediates the dissolution of the vascular basement membrane and the interstitial matrix [100]. Even though angiogenesis is the common leading cause of cancer progression and resistance to therapy, abruptly targeting the crucial contributing factor, VEGF, could potentially be risky. The TME can serve as a clonal selection niche or compensatory substance-providing source, facilitating resistance [101]. According to certain observations from human cancer studies, anti-VEGF therapy eventually results in regrowth of clonal populations with the characteristics of expressing higher compensatory factors such as VEGF, FGF, placental growth factor (PGF), and PDGF [102]. Also, more invasive cells can be selected, leading to tumor recurrence [102].

Abnormal neoplastic vessels can also lead to hypoxia, which enhances proliferation, angiogenesis, and metastasis in HCC. Increasing evidence suggests that hypoxia has profound effects on the development and evolution of the liver TME by regulating differentiation of both tumor and stromal cells. Reduced oxygen availability induces expression of hypoxia-inducible factor 1 (HIF-1), a major transcription factor that regulates the expression of several genes with critical roles in angiogenesis, immune evasion, invasion, and metastasis [103]. As expected, high levels of HIF-1 correlate with a bad prognosis in HCC [104]. Furthermore, activation of the HIF-1α-regulated glycolysis was closely related to HCC metastasis via *ENO1*, a glycolysis-related gene [105]. Finally, hypoxia can also induce β-catenin overexpression and intracellular accumulation through down-regulation of the endogenous degradation machinery [106].

Chronic exposure to hypoxia promotes epithelial-to-mesenchymal transition (EMT), migration and invasion, and resistance to chemotherapy in HCC cells [107]. Since hypoxia regulates many tumor-promoting features in HCC it is not surprising that it can also promote resistance to therapy, especially if the chosen therapy contributes to hypoxia. Thus, hypoxia caused by the antiangiogenic effects of sustained sorafenib therapy can induce HIF-1α activation, therefore limiting sorafenib efficiency [108]. Hypoxia can also induce resistance to treatment in HCC by creating an immunosuppressive microenvironment [109]. Thus, increased hypoxia results in recruitment and activation of multiple myeloid and lymphoid immune suppressor cells such as M2-type TAMs, myeloid-derived suppressor cells, and T_{REG} cells. In an independent study, hypoxia caused resistance to doxorubicin and HIF-2A inhibition enhanced the efficacy of doxorubicin in the treatment of HCC [110]. Taken together, angiogenesis may play an important role in response to therapy in HCC, underlying the importance of better understanding the effects that different therapeutics have in this process.

Concluding Remarks

Different therapies are successfully used for the clinical management of HCC, a very lethal malignancy, and several strategies have been proposed for overcoming therapy resistance in HCC. However, limited attention has been given to TME-mediated resistance mechanisms and how they might be circumvented (Fig. 1). There are currently drugs that target various aspects of the TME in clinical trials in monotherapy or in combination with standard therapies to treat cancer [111, 112].

For example, drugs that could reduce fibrosis (such TGFB1 or MET inhibitors) or revert the immunosuppressive liver TME (such as CSF-1R inhibitors) could potentially limit the emergence of resistance. An important advantage of altering the liver TME is that the target cells are genetically stable and therefore less likely to develop resistance [33]. However, the acquisition of resistance to antiangiogenic agents through activation of alternative pathways is a possibility to consider. Moreover, specific depletion of one stromal cell type within tumors can lead to a state of imbalance within the TME, thereby leading to alterations in other stromal cell populations that contribute to intrinsic or acquired resistance [6]. Further preclinical and clinical studies will be needed to assess the full potential of targeting the liver TME, alone or in combination with current therapies.

Acknowledgements The authors gratefully thank the members of the Lujambio laboratory for useful comments on the paper. AL is funded by the American Association for the Study of Liver Diseases (AASLD) Pinnacle Research Award and the Department of Defense (DoD) Career Development and Translational Team Science Awards.

Conflict of Interest The authors declare no conflict of interest.

References

1. Bataller R, Brenner DA. Liver fibrosis. J Clin Invest. 2005;115(2):209–18. doi:10.1172/JCI24282.
2. Llovet JM, Zucman-Rossi J, Pikarsky E, Sangro B, Schwartz M, Sherman M, Gores G. Hepatocellular carcinoma. Nat Rev Dis Primers. 2016;2:16018. doi:10.1038/nrdp.2016.18.
3. Seitz HK, Stickel F. Risk factors and mechanisms of hepatocarcinogenesis with special emphasis on alcohol and oxidative stress. Biol Chem. 2006;387(4):349–60. doi:10.1515/BC.2006.047.
4. Hernandez-Gea V, Toffanin S, Friedman SL, Llovet JM. Role of the microenvironment in the pathogenesis and treatment of hepatocellular carcinoma. Gastroenterology. 2013;144(3):512–27. doi:10.1053/j.gastro.2013.01.002.
5. Giannelli G, Rani B, Dituri F, Cao Y, Palasciano G. Moving towards personalised therapy in patients with hepatocellular carcinoma: the role of the microenvironment. Gut. 2014;63(10):1668–76. doi:10.1136/gutjnl-2014-307323.
6. Quail DF, Joyce JA. Microenvironmental regulation of tumor progression and metastasis. Nat Med. 2013;19(11):1423–37. doi:10.1038/nm.3394.
7. Hanahan D, Coussens LM. Accessories to the crime: functions of cells recruited to the tumor microenvironment. Cancer Cell. 2012;21(3):309–22. doi:10.1016/j.ccr.2012.02.022.
8. Llovet JM, Schwartz M, Mazzaferro V. Resection and liver transplantation for hepatocellular carcinoma. Semin Liver Dis. 2005;25(2):181–200. doi:10.1055/s-2005-871198.
9. Hoshida Y, Villanueva A, Kobayashi M, Peix J, Chiang DY, Camargo A, Gupta S, Moore J, Wrobel MJ, Lerner J, Reich M, Chan JA, Glickman JN, Ikeda K, Hashimoto M, Watanabe G, Daidone MG, Roayaie S, Schwartz M, Thung S, Salvesen HB, Gabriel S, Mazzaferro V, Bruix J, Friedman SL, Kumada H, Llovet JM, Golub TR. Gene expression in fixed tissues and outcome in hepatocellular carcinoma. N Engl J Med. 2008;359(19):1995–2004. doi:10.1056/NEJMoa0804525.
10. Bhowmick NA, Chytil A, Plieth D, Gorska AE, Dumont N, Shappell S, Washington MK, Neilson EG, Moses HL. TGF-beta signaling in fibroblasts modulates the oncogenic potential of adjacent epithelia. Science. 2004;303(5659):848–51. doi:10.1126/science.1090922.

11. Trimboli AJ, Cantemir-Stone CZ, Li F, Wallace JA, Merchant A, Creasap N, Thompson JC, Caserta E, Wang H, Chong JL, Naidu S, Wei G, Sharma SM, Stephens JA, Fernandez SA, Gurcan MN, Weinstein MB, Barsky SH, Yee L, Rosol TJ, Stromberg PC, Robinson ML, Pepin F, Hallett M, Park M, Ostrowski MC, Leone G. Pten in stromal fibroblasts suppresses mammary epithelial tumours. Nature. 2009;461(7267):1084–91. doi:10.1038/nature08486.
12. European Association for the Study of the Liver; European Organisation for Research and Treatment of Cancer. EASL-EORTC clinical practice guidelines: management of hepatocellular carcinoma. J Hepatol. 2012;56(4):908–43. doi:10.1016/j.jhep.2011.12.001.
13. Clavien PA, Lesurtel M, Bossuyt PM, Gores GJ, Langer B, Perrier A, OLT for HCC Consensus Group. Recommendations for liver transplantation for hepatocellular carcinoma: an international consensus conference report. Lancet Oncol. 2012;13(1):e11–22. doi:10.1016/S1470-2045(11)70175-9.
14. Forner A, Llovet JM, Bruix J. Hepatocellular carcinoma. Lancet. 2012;379(9822):1245–55. doi:10.1016/S0140-6736(11)61347-0.
15. Yu H, Burke CT. Comparison of percutaneous ablation technologies in the treatment of malignant liver tumors. Semin Intervent Radiol. 2014;31(2):129–37. doi:10.1055/s-0034-1373788.
16. Llovet JM, Real MI, Montana X, Planas R, Coll S, Aponte J, Ayuso C, Sala M, Muchart J, Sola R, Rodes J, Bruix J. Arterial embolisation or chemoembolisation versus symptomatic treatment in patients with unresectable hepatocellular carcinoma: a randomised controlled trial. Lancet. 2002;359(9319):1734–9. doi:10.1016/S0140-6736(02)08649-X.
17. Llovet JM, Bruix J. Systematic review of randomized trials for unresectable hepatocellular carcinoma: chemoembolization improves survival. Hepatology. 2003;37(2):429–42. doi:10.1053/jhep.2003.50047.
18. Llovet JM, Ricci S, Mazzaferro V, Hilgard P, Gane E, Blanc JF, de Oliveira AC, Santoro A, Raoul JL, Forner A, Schwartz M, Porta C, Zeuzem S, Bolondi L, Greten TF, Galle PR, Seitz JF, Borbath I, Haussinger D, Giannaris T, Shan M, Moscovici M, Voliotis D, Bruix J. Sorafenib in advanced hepatocellular carcinoma. N Engl J Med. 2008;359(4):378–90. doi:10.1056/NEJMoa0708857.
19. Wilhelm SM, Adnane L, Newell P, Villanueva A, Llovet JM, Lynch M. Preclinical overview of sorafenib, a multikinase inhibitor that targets both Raf and VEGF and PDGF receptor tyrosine kinase signaling. Mol Cancer Ther. 2008;7(10):3129–40. doi:10.1158/1535-7163.MCT-08-0013.
20. Berasain C. Hepatocellular carcinoma and sorafenib: too many resistance mechanisms? Gut. 2013;62(12):1674–5. doi:10.1136/gutjnl-2013-304564.
21. Arthur MJ. Fibrogenesis II. Metalloproteinases and their inhibitors in liver fibrosis. Am J Physiol Gastrointest Liver Physiol. 2000;279(2):G245–9.
22. Lu P, Weaver VM, Werb Z. The extracellular matrix: a dynamic niche in cancer progression. J Cell Biol. 2012;196(4):395–406. doi:10.1083/jcb.201102147.
23. Bollyky PL, Wu RP, Falk BA, Lord JD, Long SA, Preisinger A, Teng B, Holt GE, Standifer NE, Braun KR, Xie CF, Samuels PL, Vernon RB, Gebe JA, Wight TN, Nepom GT. ECM components guide IL-10 producing regulatory T-cell (TR1) induction from effector memory T-cell precursors. Proc Natl Acad Sci U S A. 2011;108(19):7938–43. doi:10.1073/pnas.1017360108.
24. Gabele E, Brenner DA, Rippe RA. Liver fibrosis: signals leading to the amplification of the fibrogenic hepatic stellate cell. Front Biosci. 2003;8:d69–77.
25. Hemmann S, Graf J, Roderfeld M, Roeb E. Expression of MMPs and TIMPs in liver fibrosis – a systematic review with special emphasis on anti-fibrotic strategies. J Hepatol. 2007;46(5):955–75. doi:10.1016/j.jhep.2007.02.003.
26. Mueller S, Sandrin L. Liver stiffness: a novel parameter for the diagnosis of liver disease. Hepat Med. 2010;2:49–67.
27. Bissell MJ, Radisky D. Putting tumours in context. Nat Rev Cancer. 2001;1(1):46–54. doi:10.1038/35094059.
28. Roskelley CD, Bissell MJ. The dominance of the microenvironment in breast and ovarian cancer. Semin Cancer Biol. 2002;12(2):97–104. doi:10.1006/scbi.2001.0417.

29. Kharaishvili G, Simkova D, Bouchalova K, Gachechiladze M, Narsia N, Bouchal J. The role of cancer-associated fibroblasts, solid stress and other microenvironmental factors in tumor progression and therapy resistance. Cancer Cell Int. 2014;14:41. doi:10.1186/1475-2867-14-41.
30. Provenzano PP, Cuevas C, Chang AE, Goel VK, Von Hoff DD, Hingorani SR. Enzymatic targeting of the stroma ablates physical barriers to treatment of pancreatic ductal adenocarcinoma. Cancer Cell. 2012;21(3):418–29. doi:10.1016/j.ccr.2012.01.007.
31. Olive KP, Jacobetz MA, Davidson CJ, Gopinathan A, McIntyre D, Honess D, Madhu B, Goldgraben MA, Caldwell ME, Allard D, Frese KK, Denicola G, Feig C, Combs C, Winter SP, Ireland-Zecchini H, Reichelt S, Howat WJ, Chang A, Dhara M, Wang L, Ruckert F, Grutzmann R, Pilarsky C, Izeradjene K, Hingorani SR, Huang P, Davies SE, Plunkett W, Egorin M, Hruban RH, Whitebread N, McGovern K, Adams J, Iacobuzio-Donahue C, Griffiths J, Tuveson DA. Inhibition of Hedgehog signaling enhances delivery of chemotherapy in a mouse model of pancreatic cancer. Science. 2009;324(5933):1457–61. doi:10.1126/science.1171362.
32. Chauhan VP, Martin JD, Liu H, Lacorre DA, Jain SR, Kozin SV, Stylianopoulos T, Mousa AS, Han X, Adstamongkonkul P, Popovic Z, Huang P, Bawendi MG, Boucher Y, Jain RK. Angiotensin inhibition enhances drug delivery and potentiates chemotherapy by decompressing tumour blood vessels. Nat Commun. 2013;4:2516. doi:10.1038/ncomms3516.
33. Barker HE, Paget JT, Khan AA, Harrington KJ. The tumour microenvironment after radiotherapy: mechanisms of resistance and recurrence. Nat Rev Cancer. 2015;15(7):409–25. doi:10.1038/nrc3958.
34. Cordes N, Seidler J, Durzok R, Geinitz H, Brakebusch C. beta1-integrin-mediated signaling essentially contributes to cell survival after radiation-induced genotoxic injury. Oncogene. 2006;25(9):1378–90. doi:10.1038/sj.onc.1209164.
35. Park CC, Zhang HJ, Yao ES, Park CJ, Bissell MJ. Beta1 integrin inhibition dramatically enhances radiotherapy efficacy in human breast cancer xenografts. Cancer Res. 2008;68(11):4398–405. doi:10.1158/0008-5472.CAN-07-6390.
36. Mantoni TS, Lunardi S, Al-Assar O, Masamune A, Brunner TB. Pancreatic stellate cells radioprotect pancreatic cancer cells through beta1-integrin signaling. Cancer Res. 2011;71(10):3453–8. doi:10.1158/0008-5472.CAN-10-1633.
37. Olson OC, Joyce JA. Cysteine cathepsin proteases: regulators of cancer progression and therapeutic response. Nat Rev Cancer. 2015;15(12):712–29. doi:10.1038/nrc4027.
38. Schrader J, Gordon-Walker TT, Aucott RL, van Deemter M, Quaas A, Walsh S, Benten D, Forbes SJ, Wells RG, Iredale JP. Matrix stiffness modulates proliferation, chemotherapeutic response, and dormancy in hepatocellular carcinoma cells. Hepatology. 2011;53(4):1192–205. doi:10.1002/hep.24108.
39. Nguyen TV, Sleiman M, Moriarty T, Herrick WG, Peyton SR. Sorafenib resistance and JNK signaling in carcinoma during extracellular matrix stiffening. Biomaterials. 2014;35(22):5749–59. doi:10.1016/j.biomaterials.2014.03.058.
40. Straussman R, Morikawa T, Shee K, Barzily-Rokni M, Qian ZR, Du J, Davis A, Mongare MM, Gould J, Frederick DT, Cooper ZA, Chapman PB, Solit DB, Ribas A, Lo RS, Flaherty KT, Ogino S, Wargo JA, Golub TR. Tumour micro-environment elicits innate resistance to RAF inhibitors through HGF secretion. Nature. 2012;487(7408):500–4. doi:10.1038/nature11183.
41. Wilson TR, Fridlyand J, Yan Y, Penuel E, Burton L, Chan E, Peng J, Lin E, Wang Y, Sosman J, Ribas A, Li J, Moffat J, Sutherlin DP, Koeppen H, Merchant M, Neve R, Settleman J. Widespread potential for growth-factor-driven resistance to anticancer kinase inhibitors. Nature. 2012;487(7408):505–9. doi:10.1038/nature11249.
42. Chen W, Wu J, Shi H, Wang Z, Zhang G, Cao Y, Jiang C, Ding Y. Hepatic stellate cell coculture enables sorafenib resistance in Huh7 cells through HGF/c-Met/Akt and Jak2/Stat3 pathways. Biomed Res Int. 2014;2014:764981. doi:10.1155/2014/764981.
43. Yu G, Jing Y, Kou X, Ye F, Gao L, Fan Q, Yang Y, Zhao Q, Li R, Wu M, Wei L. Hepatic stellate cells secreted hepatocyte growth factor contributes to the chemoresistance of hepatocellular carcinoma. PLoS One. 2013;8(9):e73312. doi:10.1371/journal.pone.0073312.

44. Mantovani A, Biswas SK, Galdiero MR, Sica A, Locati M. Macrophage plasticity and polarization in tissue repair and remodelling. J Pathol. 2013;229(2):176–85. doi:10.1002/path.4133.
45. Pollard JW. Trophic macrophages in development and disease. Nat Rev Immunol. 2009;9(4):259–70. doi:10.1038/nri2528.
46. Mosser DM, Edwards JP. Exploring the full spectrum of macrophage activation. Nat Rev Immunol. 2008;8(12):958–69. doi:10.1038/nri2448.
47. Biswas SK, Mantovani A. Macrophage plasticity and interaction with lymphocyte subsets: cancer as a paradigm. Nat Immunol. 2010;11(10):889–96. doi:10.1038/ni.1937.
48. Wang HW, Joyce JA. Alternative activation of tumor-associated macrophages by IL-4: priming for protumoral functions. Cell Cycle. 2010;9(24):4824–35.
49. Duffield JS, Forbes SJ, Constandinou CM, Clay S, Partolina M, Vuthoori S, Wu S, Lang R, Iredale JP. Selective depletion of macrophages reveals distinct, opposing roles during liver injury and repair. J Clin Invest. 2005;115(1):56–65. doi:10.1172/JCI22675.
50. Zigmond E, Samia-Grinberg S, Pasmanik-Chor M, Brazowski E, Shibolet O, Halpern Z, Varol C. Infiltrating monocyte-derived macrophages and resident Kupffer cells display different ontogeny and functions in acute liver injury. J Immunol. 2014;193(1):344–53. doi:10.4049/jimmunol.1400574.
51. Yeung WH, Lo CM, Ling CC, Qi X, Geng W, Li CX, Ng KT, Forbes SJ, Guan XY, Poon RT, Fan ST, Man K. Alternatively activated (M2) macrophages promoted tumor growth and invasiveness in hepatocellular carcinoma. J Hepatol. 2014; doi:10.1016/j.jhep.2014.10.029.
52. Dai XM, Ryan GR, Hapel AJ, Dominguez MG, Russell RG, Kapp S, Sylvestre V, Stanley ER. Targeted disruption of the mouse colony-stimulating factor 1 receptor gene results in osteopetrosis, mononuclear phagocyte deficiency, increased primitive progenitor cell frequencies, and reproductive defects. Blood. 2002;99(1):111–20.
53. Zhu XD, Zhang JB, Zhuang PY, Zhu HG, Zhang W, Xiong YQ, Wu WZ, Wang L, Tang ZY, Sun HC. High expression of macrophage colony-stimulating factor in peritumoral liver tissue is associated with poor survival after curative resection of hepatocellular carcinoma. J Clin Oncol. 2008;26(16):2707–16. doi:10.1200/JCO.2007.15.6521.
54. Chen ML, Yan BS, WC L, Chen MH, Yu SL, Yang PC, Cheng AL. Sorafenib relieves cell-intrinsic and cell-extrinsic inhibitions of effector T cells in tumor microenvironment to augment antitumor immunity. Int J Cancer. 2014;134(2):319–31. doi:10.1002/ijc.28362.
55. Hipp MM, Hilf N, Walter S, Werth D, Brauer KM, Radsak MP, Weinschenk T, Singh-Jasuja H, Brossart P. Sorafenib, but not sunitinib, affects function of dendritic cells and induction of primary immune responses. Blood. 2008;111(12):5610–20. doi:10.1182/blood-2007-02-075945.
56. Zhang QB, Sun HC, Zhang KZ, Jia QA, Bu Y, Wang M, Chai ZT, Zhang QB, Wang WQ, Kong LQ, Zhu XD, Lu L, Wu WZ, Wang L, Tang ZY. Suppression of natural killer cells by sorafenib contributes to prometastatic effects in hepatocellular carcinoma. PLoS One. 2013;8(2):e55945. doi:10.1371/journal.pone.0055945.
57. Chew V, Tow C, Huang C, Bard-Chapeau E, Copeland NG, Jenkins NA, Weber A, Lim KH, Toh HC, Heikenwalder M, Ng IO, Nardin A, Abastado JP. Toll-like receptor 3 expressing tumor parenchyma and infiltrating natural killer cells in hepatocellular carcinoma patients. J Natl Cancer Inst. 2012;104(23):1796–807. doi:10.1093/jnci/djs436.
58. Ho V, Lim TS, Lee J, Steinberg J, Szmyd R, Tham M, Yaligar J, Kaldis P, Abastado JP, Chew V. TLR3 agonist and Sorafenib combinatorial therapy promotes immune activation and controls hepatocellular carcinoma progression. Oncotarget. 2015;6(29):27252–66. doi:10.18632/oncotarget.4583.
59. Zhang W, Zhu XD, Sun HC, Xiong YQ, Zhuang PY, Xu HX, Kong LQ, Wang L, Wu WZ, Tang ZY. Depletion of tumor-associated macrophages enhances the effect of sorafenib in metastatic liver cancer models by antimetastatic and antiangiogenic effects. Clin Cancer Res. 2010;16(13):3420–30. doi:10.1158/1078-0432.CCR-09-2904.
60. Chen Y, Ramjiawan RR, Reiberger T, Ng MR, Hato T, Huang Y, Ochiai H, Kitahara S, Unan EC, Reddy TP, Fan C, Huang P, Bardeesy N, Zhu AX, Jain RK, Duda DG. CXCR4 inhibition

in tumor microenvironment facilitates anti-programmed death receptor-1 immunotherapy in sorafenib-treated hepatocellular carcinoma in mice. Hepatology. 2015;61(5):1591–602. doi:10.1002/hep.27665.
61. Sprinzl MF, Reisinger F, Puschnik A, Ringelhan M, Ackermann K, Hartmann D, Schiemann M, Weinmann A, Galle PR, Schuchmann M, Friess H, Otto G, Heikenwalder M, Protzer U. Sorafenib perpetuates cellular anticancer effector functions by modulating the crosstalk between macrophages and natural killer cells. Hepatology. 2013;57(6):2358–68. doi:10.1002/hep.26328.
62. Gabrilovich DI, Nagaraj S. Myeloid-derived suppressor cells as regulators of the immune system. Nat Rev Immunol. 2009;9(3):162–74. doi:10.1038/nri2506.
63. Cai W, Qin A, Guo P, Yan D, Hu F, Yang Q, Xu M, Fu Y, Zhou J, Tang X. Clinical significance and functional studies of myeloid-derived suppressor cells in chronic hepatitis C patients. J Clin Immunol. 2013;33(4):798–808. doi:10.1007/s10875-012-9861-2.
64. Tacke RS, Lee HC, Goh C, Courtney J, Polyak SJ, Rosen HR, Hahn YS. Myeloid suppressor cells induced by hepatitis C virus suppress T-cell responses through the production of reactive oxygen species. Hepatology. 2012;55(2):343–53. doi:10.1002/hep.24700.
65. Kapanadze T, Gamrekelashvili J, Ma C, Chan C, Zhao F, Hewitt S, Zender L, Kapoor V, Felsher DW, Manns MP, Korangy F, Greten TF. Regulation of accumulation and function of myeloid derived suppressor cells in different murine models of hepatocellular carcinoma. J Hepatol. 2013;59(5):1007–13. doi:10.1016/j.jhep.2013.06.010.
66. Xu Y, Zhao W, Xu J, Li J, Hong Z, Yin Z, Wang X. Activated hepatic stellate cells promote liver cancer by induction of myeloid-derived suppressor cells through cyclooxygenase-2. Oncotarget. 2016;7(8):8866–78. doi:10.18632/oncotarget.6839.
67. Gauttier V, Judor JP, Le Guen V, Cany J, Ferry N, Conchon S. Agonistic anti-CD137 antibody treatment leads to antitumor response in mice with liver cancer. Int J Cancer. 2014;135(12):2857–67. doi:10.1002/ijc.28943.
68. Mizukoshi E, Yamashita T, Arai K, Terashima T, Kitahara M, Nakagawa H, Iida N, Fushimi K, Kaneko S. Myeloid-derived suppressor cells correlate with patient outcomes in hepatic arterial infusion chemotherapy for hepatocellular carcinoma. Cancer Immunol Immunother. 2016;65(6):715–25. doi:10.1007/s00262-016-1837-2.
69. Wang D, An G, Xie S, Yao Y, Feng G. The clinical and prognostic significance of CD14HLA-DR myeloid-derived suppressor cells in hepatocellular carcinoma patients receiving radiotherapy. Tumour Biol. 2016; doi:10.1007/s13277-016-4916-2.
70. Gao B, Jeong WI, Tian Z. Liver: an organ with predominant innate immunity. Hepatology. 2008;47(2):729–36. doi:10.1002/hep.22034.
71. Tai LH, Tanese de Souza C, Belanger S, Ly L, Alkayyal AA, Zhang J, Rintoul JL, Ananth AA, Lam T, Breitbach CJ, Falls TJ, Kirn DH, Bell JC, Makrigiannis AP, Auer RA. Preventing post-operative metastatic disease by inhibiting surgery-induced dysfunction in natural killer cells. Cancer Res. 2012; doi:10.1158/0008-5472.CAN-12-1993.
72. Jinushi M, Takehara T, Tatsumi T, Hiramatsu N, Sakamori R, Yamaguchi S, Hayashi N. Impairment of natural killer cell and dendritic cell functions by the soluble form of MHC class I-related chain A in advanced human hepatocellular carcinomas. J Hepatol. 2005;43(6):1013–20. doi:10.1016/j.jhep.2005.05.026.
73. Chuang WL, Liu HW, Chang WY. Natural killer cell activity in patients with hepatocellular carcinoma relative to early development and tumor invasion. Cancer. 1990;65(4):926–30.
74. Hoechst B, Voigtlaender T, Ormandy L, Gamrekelashvili J, Zhao F, Wedemeyer H, Lehner F, Manns MP, Greten TF, Korangy F. Myeloid derived suppressor cells inhibit natural killer cells in patients with hepatocellular carcinoma via the NKp30 receptor. Hepatology. 2009;50(3):799–807. doi:10.1002/hep.23054.
75. Wang Y, Li H, Liang Q, Liu B, Mei X, Ma Y. Combinatorial immunotherapy of sorafenib and blockade of programmed death-ligand 1 induces effective natural killer cell responses against hepatocellular carcinoma. Tumour Biol. 2015;36(3):1561–6. doi:10.1007/s13277-014-2722-2.

76. Lee WC, Wu TJ, Chou HS, Yu MC, Hsu PY, Hsu HY, Wang CC. The impact of CD4+ CD25+ T cells in the tumor microenvironment of hepatocellular carcinoma. Surgery. 2012;151(2):213–22. doi:10.1016/j.surg.2011.07.029.
77. Fu J, Xu D, Liu Z, Shi M, Zhao P, Fu B, Zhang Z, Yang H, Zhang H, Zhou C, Yao J, Jin L, Wang H, Yang Y, YX F, Wang FS. Increased regulatory T cells correlate with CD8 T-cell impairment and poor survival in hepatocellular carcinoma patients. Gastroenterology. 2007;132(7):2328–39. doi:10.1053/j.gastro.2007.03.102.
78. Unitt E, Rushbrook SM, Marshall A, Davies S, Gibbs P, Morris LS, Coleman N, Alexander GJ. Compromised lymphocytes infiltrate hepatocellular carcinoma: the role of T-regulatory cells. Hepatology. 2005;41(4):722–30. doi:10.1002/hep.20644.
79. Ormandy LA, Hillemann T, Wedemeyer H, Manns MP, Greten TF, Korangy F. Increased populations of regulatory T cells in peripheral blood of patients with hepatocellular carcinoma. Cancer Res. 2005;65(6):2457–64. doi:10.1158/0008-5472.CAN-04-3232.
80. Bates GJ, Fox SB, Han C, Leek RD, Garcia JF, Harris AL, Banham AH. Quantification of regulatory T cells enables the identification of high-risk breast cancer patients and those at risk of late relapse. J Clin Oncol. 2006;24(34):5373–80. doi:10.1200/JCO.2006.05.9584.
81. Zhou S, Chen L, Qin J, Li R, Tao H, Zhen Z, Chen H, Chen G, Yang Y, Liu B, She Z, Zhong C, Liang C. Depletion of CD4+ CD25+ regulatory T cells promotes CCL21-mediated antitumor immunity. PLoS One. 2013;8(9):e73952. doi:10.1371/journal.pone.0073952.
82. Li CX, Ling CC, Shao Y, Xu A, Li XC, Ng KT, Liu XB, Ma YY, Qi X, Liu H, Liu J, Yeung OW, Yang XX, Liu QS, Lam YF, Zhai Y, Lo CM, Man K. CXCL10/CXCR3 signaling mobilized-regulatory T cells promote liver tumor recurrence after transplantation. J Hepatol. 2016; doi:10.1016/j.jhep.2016.05.032.
83. Fu J, Zhang Z, Zhou L, Qi Z, Xing S, Lv J, Shi J, Fu B, Liu Z, Zhang JY, Jin L, Zhao Y, Lau GK, Zhao J, Wang FS. Impairment of CD4+ cytotoxic T cells predicts poor survival and high recurrence rates in patients with hepatocellular carcinoma. Hepatology. 2013;58(1):139–49. doi:10.1002/hep.26054.
84. Jia Y, Zeng Z, Li Y, Li Z, Jin L, Zhang Z, Wang L, Wang FS. Impaired function of CD4+ T follicular helper (Tfh) cells associated with hepatocellular carcinoma progression. PLoS One. 2015;10(2):e0117458. doi:10.1371/journal.pone.0117458.
85. Confer BD, Choudhary M, Lopez R, Zein NN. Monitoring serial CD4(+) T-cell function after liver transplantation can be used to predict hepatocellular carcinoma recurrence. Transplant Proc. 2015;47(1):217–22. doi:10.1016/j.transproceed.2014.10.044.
86. Cabrera R, Ararat M, Xu Y, Brusko T, Wasserfall C, Atkinson MA, Chang LJ, Liu C, Nelson DR. Immune modulation of effector CD4+ and regulatory T cell function by sorafenib in patients with hepatocellular carcinoma. Cancer Immunol Immunother. 2013;62(4):737–46. doi:10.1007/s00262-012-1380-8.
87. Gabrielson A, Wu Y, Wang H, Jiang J, Kallakury B, Gatalica Z, Reddy S, Kleiner D, Fishbein T, Johnson L, Island E, Satoskar R, Banovac F, Jha R, Kachhela J, Feng P, Zhang T, Tesfaye A, Prins P, Loffredo C, Marshall J, Weiner L, Atkins M, He AR. Intratumoral CD3 and CD8 T-cell densities associated with relapse-free survival in HCC. Cancer Immunol Res. 2016;4(5):419–30. doi:10.1158/2326-6066.CIR-15-0110.
88. Joyce JA, Fearon DT. T cell exclusion, immune privilege, and the tumor microenvironment. Science. 2015;348(6230):74–80. doi:10.1126/science.aaa6204.
89. Lim TS, Chew V, Sieow JL, Goh S, Yeong JP, Soon AL, Ricciardi-Castagnoli P. PD-1 expression on dendritic cells suppresses CD8 T cell function and antitumor immunity. Oncoimmunology. 2016;5(3):e1085146. doi:10.1080/2162402X.2015.1085146.
90. Chen J, Ji T, Zhao J, Li G, Zhang J, Jin R, Liu J, Liu X, Liang X, Huang D, Xie A, Lin H, Cang Y, Cai X. Sorafenib-resistant hepatocellular carcinoma stratified by phosphorylated ERK activates PD-1 immune checkpoint. Oncotarget. 2016; doi:10.18632/oncotarget.8978.
91. Tredan O, Galmarini CM, Patel K, Tannock IF. Drug resistance and the solid tumor microenvironment. J Natl Cancer Inst. 2007;99(19):1441–54. doi:10.1093/jnci/djm135.

92. Jain RK. Determinants of tumor blood flow: a review. Cancer Res. 1988;48(10):2641–58.
93. Sevick EM, Jain RK. Geometric resistance to blood flow in solid tumors perfused ex vivo: effects of tumor size and perfusion pressure. Cancer Res. 1989;49(13):3506–12.
94. Padera TP, Stoll BR, Tooredman JB, Capen D, di Tomaso E, Jain RK. Pathology: cancer cells compress intratumour vessels. Nature. 2004;427(6976):695. doi:10.1038/427695a.
95. Durand RE. Intermittent blood flow in solid tumours--an under-appreciated source of 'drug resistance'. Cancer Metastasis Rev. 2001;20(1-2):57–61.
96. Xiong YQ, Sun HC, Zhang W, Zhu XD, Zhuang PY, Zhang JB, Wang L, Wu WZ, Qin LX, Tang ZY. Human hepatocellular carcinoma tumor-derived endothelial cells manifest increased angiogenesis capability and drug resistance compared with normal endothelial cells. Clin Cancer Res. 2009;15(15):4838–46. doi:10.1158/1078-0432.CCR-08-2780.
97. Bergers G, Benjamin LE. Tumorigenesis and the angiogenic switch. Nat Rev Cancer. 2003;3(6):401–10. doi:10.1038/nrc1093.
98. Kuczynski EA, Yin M, Bar-Zion A, Lee CR, Butz H, Man S, Daley F, Vermeulen PB, Yousef GM, Foster FS, Reynolds AR, Kerbel RS. Co-option of liver vessels and not sprouting angiogenesis drives acquired sorafenib resistance in hepatocellular carcinoma. J Natl Cancer Inst. 2016;108(8). doi:10.1093/jnci/djw030.
99. Lichtenberger BM, Tan PK, Niederleithner H, Ferrara N, Petzelbauer P, Sibilia M. Autocrine VEGF signaling synergizes with EGFR in tumor cells to promote epithelial cancer development. Cell. 2010;140(2):268–79. doi:10.1016/j.cell.2009.12.046.
100. Zhu AX, Duda DG, Sahani DV, Jain RK. HCC and angiogenesis: possible targets and future directions. Nat Rev Clin Oncol. 2011;8(5):292–301. doi:10.1038/nrclinonc.2011.30.
101. Tsai MJ, Chang WA, Huang MS, Kuo PL. Tumor microenvironment: a new treatment target for cancer. ISRN Biochem. 2014;2014:351959. doi:10.1155/2014/351959.
102. Bottsford-Miller JN, Coleman RL, Sood AK. Resistance and escape from antiangiogenesis therapy: clinical implications and future strategies. J Clin Oncol. 2012;30(32):4026–34. doi:10.1200/JCO.2012.41.9242.
103. Semenza GL. Oxygen sensing, homeostasis, and disease. N Engl J Med. 2011;365(6):537–47. doi:10.1056/NEJMra1011165.
104. Wu XZ, Xie GR, Chen D. Hypoxia and hepatocellular carcinoma: the therapeutic target for hepatocellular carcinoma. J Gastroenterol Hepatol. 2007;22(8):1178–82. doi:10.1111/j.1440-1746.2007.04997.x.
105. Hamaguchi T, Iizuka N, Tsunedomi R, Hamamoto Y, Miyamoto T, Iida M, Tokuhisa Y, Sakamoto K, Takashima M, Tamesa T, Oka M. Glycolysis module activated by hypoxia-inducible factor 1alpha is related to the aggressive phenotype of hepatocellular carcinoma. Int J Oncol. 2008;33(4):725–31.
106. Liu L, Zhu XD, Wang WQ, Shen Y, Qin Y, Ren ZG, Sun HC, Tang ZY. Activation of beta-catenin by hypoxia in hepatocellular carcinoma contributes to enhanced metastatic potential and poor prognosis. Clin Cancer Res. 2010;16(10):2740–50. doi:10.1158/1078-0432.CCR-09-2610.
107. Jiao M, Nan KJ. Activation of PI3 kinase/Akt/HIF-1alpha pathway contributes to hypoxia-induced epithelial-mesenchymal transition and chemoresistance in hepatocellular carcinoma. Int J Oncol. 2012;40(2):461–8. doi:10.3892/ijo.2011.1197.
108. Liang Y, Zheng T, Song R, Wang J, Yin D, Wang L, Liu H, Tian L, Fang X, Meng X, Jiang H, Liu J, Liu L. Hypoxia-mediated sorafenib resistance can be overcome by EF24 through Von Hippel-Lindau tumor suppressor-dependent HIF-1alpha inhibition in hepatocellular carcinoma. Hepatology. 2013;57(5):1847–57. doi:10.1002/hep.26224.
109. Flecken T, Schmidt N, Hild S, Gostick E, Drognitz O, Zeiser R, Schemmer P, Bruns H, Eiermann T, Price DA, Blum HE, Neumann-Haefelin C, Thimme R. Immunodominance and functional alterations of tumor-associated antigen-specific CD8+ T-cell responses in hepatocellular carcinoma. Hepatology. 2014;59(4):1415–26. doi:10.1002/hep.26731.
110. He C, Sun XP, Qiao H, Jiang X, Wang D, Jin X, Dong X, Wang J, Jiang H, Sun X. Downregulating hypoxia-inducible factor-2alpha improves the efficacy of doxoru-

bicin in the treatment of hepatocellular carcinoma. Cancer Sci. 2012;103(3):528–34. doi:10.1111/j.1349-7006.2011.02177.x.

111. Melero I, Berman DM, Aznar MA, Korman AJ, Gracia JL, Haanen J. Evolving synergistic combinations of targeted immunotherapies to combat cancer. Nat Rev Cancer. 2015;15(8):457–72. doi:10.1038/nrc3973.

112. Sanmamed MF, Chester C, Melero I, Kohrt H. Defining the optimal murine models to investigate immune checkpoint blockers and their combination with other immunotherapies. Ann Oncol. 2016; doi:10.1093/annonc/mdw041.

Contribution of the Cancer Stem Cell Phenotype to Hepatocellular Carcinoma Resistance

Darko Castven, Carolin Czauderna, and Jens U. Marquardt

Abstract The cancer stem cell (CSC) hypothesis is an increasingly accepted concept in cancer research that provides a plausible explanation for the considerable phenotypic and molecular heterogeneities observed in hepatocellular carcinoma (HCC) which hampers therapeutic progress. The hypothesis infers that CSCs share functional properties similar to adult stem cells, such as self-renewal and differentiation capacity, and are exclusively responsible for tumor evolution. By definition, CSCs are held responsible not only for tumor initiation and progression but also acquisition of chemoresistance and the fueling of relapse after therapy. Therefore, the CSC model has significant implications both for translational research as well as clinical applications, in particular for the development of novel treatment strategies. Implicit in the concept is the need for therapeutic targeting of CSCs to effectively diminish tumor growth. Therefore, a better understanding of the molecular mechanisms that lead to induction of stemness and drive CSCs in HCC is of crucial importance. In this chapter, we aim to highlight important aspects of the CSC biology in the context of clinical and therapeutic progress. Besides a critical reflection of the cellular origin of CSCs, this will also include discussion on the importance of the diseased hepatic microenvironment for oncogenic reprogramming and induction of stemness in HCC. Moreover, we will highlight the relevance of CSC markers as diagnostic and/or predictive biomarkers. Most importantly, we will delineate the potential of therapeutic targeting of CSCs to overcome therapeutic resistance and improve the HCC patients' outcome.

Darko Castven and Carolin Czauderna contributed equally to this work.

D. Castven • C. Czauderna • J.U. Marquardt (✉)
Department of Medicine I, Lichtenberg Research Group for Molecular Hepatocarcinogenesis, Johannes Gutenberg University, Mainz, Germany
e-mail: marquarj@uni-mainz.de

A. Villanueva (ed.), *Resistance to Molecular Therapies for Hepatocellular Carcinoma*, Resistance to Targeted Anti-Cancer Therapeutics,
DOI 10.1007/978-3-319-56197-4_4

Keywords Cancer stem cells • Tumor-initiating cells • Acquired resistance • Cell-of-origin • Oncogenic reprogramming • Microenvironment • Stemness

Abbreviations

ABC	Adenosine triphosphate (ATP)-binding cassette
ABCG2	Adenosine triphosphate (ATP)-binding cassette G2
AFP	Alpha-fetoprotein
AKT	AKT8 virus oncogene cellular homolog
BCL-2	B-cell lymphoma 2
BEC	Biliary epithelial cell
CD13	Cluster of differentiation 13; aminopeptidase N
CD133	Cluster of differentiation 133; prominin 1
CD24	Cluster of differentiation 24; mucin-like cell surface glycoprotein; heat stable antigen
CD44	Cluster of differentiation 44
CD45	Cluster of differentiation 45; leucocyte common antigen
CD90	Cluster of differentiation 90; thymus cell antigen
c-Kit	Tyrosine-protein kinase Kit
CSC	Cancer stem cell
CUDR	Long noncoding RNA cancer upregulated drug resistant
DCP	Des-gamma-carboxy prothrombin
DNA	Deoxyribonucleic acid
DNMT1	DNA methyltransferase 1
EGFR	Epidermal growth factor receptor
EMT	Epithelial–mesenchymal transition
EpCAM	Epithelial cell adhesion molecule
FGF	Fibroblast growth factor
GP73	Golgi protein-73
HCC	Hepatocellular carcinoma
HDAC	Histone deacetylases

Introduction

The traditional model of carcinogenesis suggests a clonal evolution as the origin of tumor formation. According to this model cancer arises as the consequence of stochastic genetic events that can be induced in any cell of a tissue. In contrast, the cancer stem cell (CSC) model postulates that a single CSC promotes a hierarchic organization within tumors [1]. These CSCs comprise only a subfraction of the tumor cells (<1%) and rest on the apex of tumor formation. By definition, CSCs are exclusively responsible to drive tumor initiation, progression as well as tumor heterogeneity. Although the existence of stem-like tumor cells that harbor the ability to generate tumors in vitro and in vivo is not new, increasing interest and compelling evidence for CSCs in solid tumors only emerged in the last decade [2–6]. However, while the CSC and the stochastic models have fundamental conceptual differences, it is worth mentioning that both models are not mutually exclusive. Current findings even favor a likelihood of complementary co-existence of both models based on the assumption that cancer is a genetically generated disease that is maintained and tightly regulated by epigenetic changes [7].

According to the model, CSCs possess unlimited proliferative and high metastatic properties. In addition, the CSCs are characterized by high activity of multidrug resistance transporters, i.e. confer to chemoresistance, which places these cells in the focus of translational research [8]. The CSC concept has several important clinical implications that include diagnosis, prevention and, most importantly, therapy. Classical chemotherapeutic compounds are designed to predominantly target highly proliferative cells, which are unlikely to be CSCs. Similarly, since tumor relapse as well as therapy resistance are frequently observed during molecular targeted-therapies these treatment strategies might also miss the CSCs (Fig. 1) [9–13]. Therefore, for successful eradication of tumors that follow a hierarchic organization, the development of new treatment approaches directed towards the CSCs seems necessary. This implies a more detailed understanding of the molecular alterations that contribute to fundamental CSC properties such as self-renewal, differentiation, seeding of metastasis and chemoresistance. The identification and characterization of these stemness pathways and molecules might help to identify common CSC-targets and complement existing therapies.

The Cellular Origin of Hepatic Cancer Stem Cells

In normal tissues phenotypic diversity is derived and maintained by adult tissue stem cells [14]. In analogy, the CSC model is helpful to explain cancer heterogeneity that is observed within many clonally-derived tumors including HCC [5, 15–18]. However, despite similarity in functional properties between CSC and normal tissue stem cells resembling self-renewal and differentiation capacity, the term CSC does not refer to the putative cellular origin but rather key stemness characteristics intrinsic for both cell types [19]. Nevertheless, determination of the cellular origin is of great translational value and different scenarios need to be considered to define the origins of CSCs and the resulting tumor heterogeneity [5, 8]: (1) Differentiation arrest of adult tissue stem cells and/or progenitor cells, (2) dedifferentiation of mature cells, and, less likely, (3) trans-differentiation of stem cells from different tissues, e.g. bone marrow. A combination of all three possibilities within a tumor would be another conceivable explanation (Fig. 2) [20].

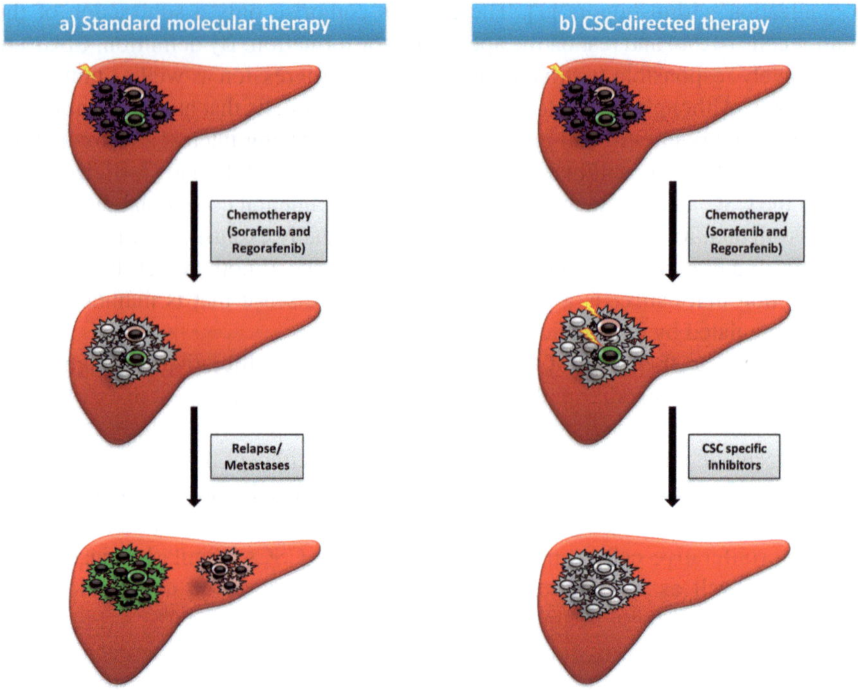

Fig. 1 Targeting of the tumor cells. (**a**) Standard molecular therapy is supposed to eradicate only the bulk of differentiated tumor cells, while CSCs, that harbor a higher chemoresistance potential, are left unharmed. Therefore, relapse and metastases formation is frequently observed after treatment with conventional and/or targeted chemotherapy; (**b**) In contrast, therapies that specifically target (cancer-) stemness might complement classical therapies and yield to a sustained anti-tumor response

The relative contribution of each postulated cellular origin is also highly impaired by the type of liver injury, signals from the diseased liver microenvironment, and the contributing mutagen(s). Over the last years, the cellular origin of HCC and detailed molecular mechanisms driving cancer stemness are the focus of great interest for cancer research and, in the end, have broad clinical implications [21, 22]. While successful early diagnosis would aim for biomarkers that specifically detect CSCs and early signs of malignant transformation, the identification of the cellular origin of CSC ("cell-at-risk") would be required to reduce the number of CSCs effectively, i.e., in CSC-directed therapies. Although many common oncogenic pathways are activated in human HCC, considerable redundancy in the activation of these pathways during regeneration and carcinogenesis impairs effective targeting of CSCs [22, 23]. Therefore, a detailed understanding of the cellular origin in liver cancer is of critical importance and required to improve the limited therapeutic options for HCC. A long life span coupled with strong regenerative potential make mature hepatocytes a prime target for malignant transformation alongside chronic liver diseases [14]. However, many of these diseases as well as pre-neoplastic stages of hepatocarcinogenesis display activation of markers frequently associated with

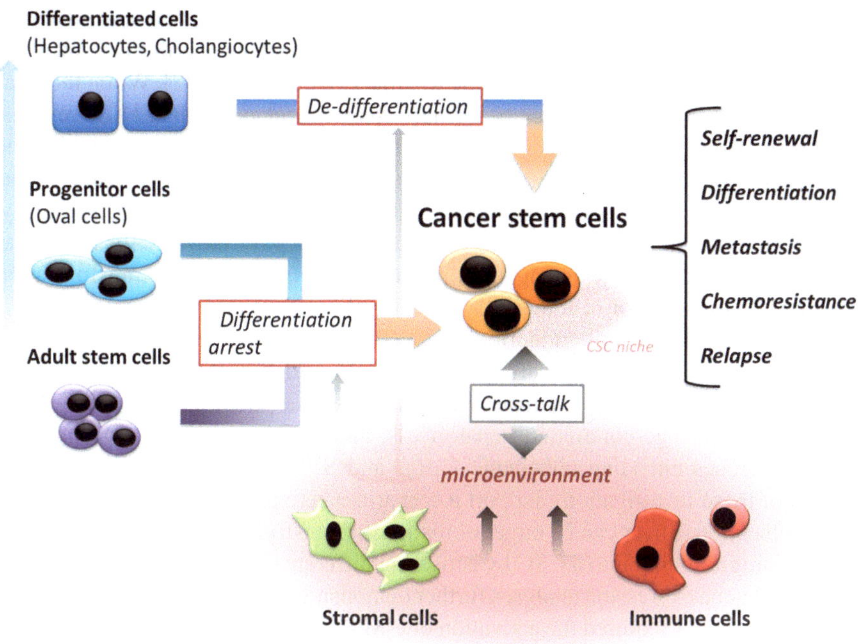

Fig. 2 Cellular origins of CSCs. Different scenarios might be important for the generation of CSCs in HCC. CSCs might originate through de-differentiation of mature hepatocytes or through differentiation arrest of stem/progenitor cells. Alternatively, both mechanisms could potentially induce stemness-features in HCC, thereby contributing to liver tumor heterogeneity. The transformation of the cell of origin to a CSC might be defined by the acquisition of stemness as well as tumorigenic features. This process is highly dependent on the type of liver injury and driven by signals from the diseased liver microenvironment

stemness traits, thus, raising a possibility of stem/progenitor cell origin of liver cancer [24, 25]. Interesting investigations recently demonstrated that hepatic stem/progenitor cell origin of liver cancer when introduced in a pre-existing chronic liver damage with compensatory hepatocyte proliferation [26]. Additionally, different whole genome analyses clearly showed that adverse clinical features and a particular poor clinical outcome characterize HCC which harbors a progenitor-cell origin [27–29]. Nevertheless, the concept of progenitor-cell origin of HCC is not undebated and other studies show that hepatocarcinogenesis might be predominantly driven by transformation of hepatocytes [30]. The latter case would also implicate that the identified molecular profiles of human HCCs resembling stem/progenitor cells may simply reflect the acquisition of the stem-like traits in hepatocyte-derived tumors rather than their progenitor cell origin. These observations would also indicate that cellular plasticity is a hallmark feature of HCC. In line with this, not all hepatocytes seem to contribute to the HCC development [31]. Therefore, it is crucial to determine the exact location, properties and molecular stimuli leading to their transformation [31].

Several lines of evidence further indicate that hepatocytes can undergo hepatocyte-to-BEC (biliary epithelial cells) reprogramming in response to acute and chronic biliary injury, and give rise to biliary tract cancers [32]. While the relative contribution of hepatocytes to primary liver cancer other than HCC remains unclear and may only represent rare events, these observations demonstrate that the oncogenic potential of hepatocytes is highly context-dependent and likely stems from the oncogenic field-effect determined by the type of hepatic injury. Understanding the cellular origin of liver cancer will pave the way for molecular dissection of the specific oncogenic programs driving hepatocyte transformation and the identification of new therapeutic and/or diagnostic targets.

To address the contribution of different cell types for hepatocarcinogenesis, Holczbauer et al. recently investigated the capacity of different hepatic lineage cells to acquire CSC properties by using transduced mouse primary hepatic progenitor cells (HPC), lineage-committed hepatoblasts, and differentiated adult hepatocytes with transgenes encoding oncogenic H-Ras and SV-40 large T-antigen [33]. The results of these investigations support a scenario where all different hepatic lineage cells in the mouse liver can be target of malignant transformation and undergo oncogenic reprogramming into a CSC by activating different cell type-specific pathways. Integrated gene expression analyses further demonstrate that transformation of hepatocytes into CSCs required the activation of c-MYC and its target genes. Conversely, stable knockdown of c-MYC in transformed adult hepatocytes reduced both the CSC properties as well as the in vivo tumorigenicity. To further support a causative role of MYC during malignant transformation in HCC and for the biology of hepatic CSCs, Akita et al. tested the effect of distinct levels of c-MYC overexpression by using two dose-dependent tetracycline-inducible systems in different hepatoma cell lines [34]. The authors could demonstrate that c-MYC expression levels have a differential impact on liver CSC characteristics. At low levels, c-MYC activation led to increased proliferation and enhanced CSC properties. However, when exceeding a threshold level, c-MYC induced a pro-apoptotic program and, subsequently, a loss of CSC potential both in vitro and in vivo. Mechanistically, c-MYC-induced self-renewal capacity of liver cancer cells was exerted in a p53-dependent manner. In summary, our results established c-MYC as a master regulator and gatekeeper for the CSC phenotype in liver cancer cells. However, regardless of the cellular origin and the corresponding activated oncogenic programs, acquisition of stemness seems to be required to induce HCC development [35, 36]. The significance of this oncogenic reprogramming for HCC development supports the notion that targeting the stemness traits may provide an effective therapeutic strategy for liver cancer [35, 37, 38].

The Importance of the Hepatic Microenvironment for Induction of a Cancer Stem Cell Phenotype

HCCs commonly develop in chronically damaged liver tissues resulting from chronic regenerative and inflammatory processes that generate an adverse microenvironment, thereby, promoting tumor initiation and progression [39]. Expansion of cancer cells with stemness features is commonly observed during this process supporting a putative progenitor cell origin in liver cancer. While the CSC hypothesis provides a plausible explanation for the observed phenotypic heterogeneity of hepatocellular cancers, detailed information on the prognostic relevance of CSCs is missing. The importance of the cellular localization of putative CSCs is further supported by recent investigations demonstrating the existence of stem-like cells within the surgical margin of HCC that predicted rapid recurrence [40]. Furthermore, the significant impact of the tumor microenvironment for the outcome of HCC patients supports a potential cross-talk between CSCs and stromal cells that could possibly lead to novel therapeutic approaches [41]. In support of this finding, genomic analyses provided evidence that genetic profiles with significant association to clinical features can be generated from the surrounding non-tumor liver tissue, whereas gene-expression profiles of tumor tissue failed to yield significant association with survival [41].

Important pro-inflammatory and pro-oncogenic effects seem to be associated with activation of IL-6 and nuclear factor κB (NF-κB) signaling in the liver. Notably, both pathways are prominent members of dominant signaling pathways involved in the so-called inflammation-fibrosis-cancer axis and are commonly disrupted during the majority of inflammatory chronic liver diseases [42, 43]. While the key role of NF-κB activation during multi-stage hepatocarcinogenesis is well documented, the absence of NF-κB by genetic loss of the regulatory NF-κB subunit *NEMO* in hepatocytes also promoted liver cancer development [39]. These investigations underline recent observations that alterations of oncogenic molecules in liver cancer are context and cell type dependent [44]. The oncogenic response is most likely determined by the type of liver injury and the cellular target of malignant transformation. Nevertheless, our previous investigations on hepatic CSCs demonstrated that epigenetic modulation increased the frequency of cells with CSC properties within prospectively isolated human hepatoma cells as judged by self-renewal, superior tumor-initiating capacity in serial transplantations, and direct cell tracking experiments [45]. When we applied integrative transcriptome analysis to prospectively isolated hepatic CSCs, we demonstrated that stemness-associated gene sets are commonly activated by distinct oncogenic pathways (e.g., EGFR, SRC, and MYC) in individual tumors. Consistently, a commonly altered key pathway was an activation of NF-κB signaling [46].

To investigate whether NF-κB could be a potential target for a CSCs-directed therapy in liver cancer, we inhibited NF-κB signaling in several hepatoma cells and freshly isolated liver cancer cells by using curcumin, an effective IKK inhibitor, RNAi against p65 and selective peptide SN50 with the overall goal to evaluate the effect of NF-κB inhibition on the frequency and functional properties of putative liver TICs in order to define the molecular mechanisms underlying the CSC-depletion. We could demonstrate that inhibition of NF-κB effectively diminished stemness features in a subgroup of liver cancer cells by NF-κB-mediated inhibition of histone deacetylases (HDACs). Consistently, co-administration of a class I and II HDAC inhibitors sensitized the curcumin-resistant cells to curcumin treatment. Further, integration of a predictive signature with our HCC database indicated that

HCCs with progenitor cell features are most likely to be sensitive to NF-κB inhibition. Specific interference with the inflammatory pathways in the liver such as NF-κB might, therefore, be a promising therapeutic strategy for HCCs that share stemness features [47]. A recent study aimed at the characterization of molecules with relevance for homeostasis of a specific CSC niche in the hepatic microenvironment. The authors identified laminin-332 as a crucial component of this niche and demonstrated that targeting of the molecule might diminish stemness potential, effectively reduce the frequency of CSCs and help to overcome therapeutic resistance in liver cancer [48].

In summary, the above-mentioned studies clearly show the crucial importance of the diseased hepatic microenvironment for the induction and maintenance of stemness properties. This specific niche preserves phenotypic plasticity, protects from immune-surveillance, facilitates metastatic spread and contributes to chemoresistance of hepatic CSCs [49]. Therefore, targeting of the cross-talk between CSCs and cells of the microenvironment seems to be a promising strategy.

Identification of Cancer Stem Cells and Clinical Relevance of Cancer Stem Cell Markers in Liver Cancer

Early detection and surveillance of HCC relies on imaging (e.g. by ultrasound) and serological markers such as AFP, AFP-L3, des-gamma-carboxy prothrombin (DCP), golgi protein-73 (GP73), osteopontin (OPN) and others [50]. However, half of HCC patients present with normal or only slightly elevated AFP serum levels at time of diagnosis [51]. Thus, there is an urgent need for novel molecular diagnostic, predictive and therapeutic biomarkers. In this context, the prognostic relevance of CSC markers, suggested by different studies, might become particularly important [52]. Current approaches for the isolation of CSCs rely on surrogate markers and/or functional properties of the cells, i.e. cell surface markers (mainly adapted from hematopoietic and adult tissue stem cells), or surrogate characteristics such as anchorage independent growth, chemo-resistance, self-renewal, asymmetric division and pluripotency [1]. Antigen-based approaches utilize different cell surface markers whereas functional isolation relies on the described surrogate characteristics. The latter approaches are particularly useful when the specific CSC markers have not been clearly defined.

Given the plasticity of the CSCs, it is unlikely that CSCs can be defined by a single marker or a single functional property. For these reasons, combinations of functional and antigenic approaches seem most appropriate for the identification and isolation of hepatic CSCs [15, 29, 53, 54]. Recent studies further showed that the different identified CSC markers could be useful as prognostic biomarkers and in predicting tumor recurrence and drug sensitivity [52]. Additionally, key signaling pathways for sustaining cancer-stemness could also provide new therapeutic strategies to overcome chemoresistance. The following paragraphs will outline important clinical associations of most frequently used CSC markers in HCC (Table 1).

Table 1 CSC marker in hepatocellular carcinoma

CSC marker	Cell line and tumorigenicity		Molecular mechanisms	Clinical characteristics	References
EpCAM	Huh1, Huh7	2×10^2	Wnt/beta-catenin signaling	Tumorigenicity, chemoresistance, tumor relapse, poor prognosis	[26, 56, 75, 105, 120, 121]
	PLC/PRF/5, Li-7	1×10^2			
	Primary HCC	1×10^4			
CD133	Huh7	1×10^3	AKT/PKB signaling; HIF-1α; MAPK/PI3K; neurotensin/IL-8/CXCL1; drug-efflux transporter	Tumorigenicity, chemo-/radioresistance, prognosis, vascular invasion, early recurrence	[17, 53, 61, 84–86, 89]
	PLC8024	5×10^4			
	SMMC-7221	1×10^2			
CD90	Huh7, MHCC97L, MHCC97H, HepG2, Hep3B	5×10^2	Not known	Tumorigenicity, circulating CSCs	[52, 54]
	Primary HCC	2.5×10^3			
	Blood samples	1×10^4			
CD44	SMMC-7221, MHCC-LM3, MHCC-97L	1×10^2	Regulation of TGF-β signaling	Tumorigenicity, chemoresistance, invasion, metastasis	[89, 128]
CD24	PLC/PRF/5, HLE	5×10^2	STAT3-mediated NANOG regulation	Tumorigenicity, chemoresistance, metastasis, tumor relapse	[73, 96]
	Primary HCC	4×10^3			
CD13	Huh7, PLC/PRF/5	1×10^2	Regulation of redox status	Tumorigenicity, chemoresistance, tumor relapse	[98]
OV6	Huh7, PLC, SMMC7721, Hep3B, HepG2	5×10^3	Wnt/beta-catenin signaling	Tumorigenicity, chemoresistance, invasion, metastasis	[52, 99]
SP cells	HCCLM3, MHCC97-H, MHCC97-L, Hep3B	2×10^3	Different stemness pathways	Tumorigenicity, chemoresistance, tumor relapse, prognosis	[15, 45, 101, 102]
	Huh7, PLC/PRF/5, WRL68, KMCH	1×10^3			

EpCAM (Epithelial cell adhesion molecule; CD326) is an onco-fetal transmembrane glycoprotein belonging to a family of adhesion molecules. EpCAM is expressed in almost all carcinomas, embryonic liver tissue, bile duct epithelium as well as in proliferating bile ductules of a cirrhotic liver; but absent on hepatocytes [55, 74]. Yamashita et al. reported that EpCAM could be used as a CSC marker for HCC. Consistently, EpCAM+ hepatoma cells as well as primary EpCAM+/AFP+ HCC cells showed superior tumor-initiation capacity in NOD/SCID mice compared to their EpCAM- counterparts [29]. In addition to the high tumorigenic potential, prospectively isolated EpCAM+ cells possessed CSC-like characteristics as well as chemoresistance against traditional chemotherapeutic compounds such as doxorubicin and 5-Fluoruracil. Further, high levels of EpCAM expression in HCC have been associated with poor overall survival. Based on these results, Yamashita et al. proposed a new prognostic classification system and classified HCC patients into four subgroups depending on the expression of EpCAM and AFP. Notably, the subgroup with highest levels of both genes HCC (i.e. EpCAM+/AFP+) showed high activation of stemness markers and possessed the worst prognosis [56]. Moreover, targeting of EpCAM by RNA interference significantly decreased CSC frequency and reduced both tumorigenicity as well as invasive properties of hepatic CSCs [29]. Since EpCAM is supposed to be a WNT/β-Catenin target gene, Wnt signaling inhibitors could improve the sensitivity to treatment of EpCAM+ HCC [75]. However, given the high redundancy of the WNT pathway members, WNT-inhibitor based approaches still requires experimental and clinical validation. From the diagnostic point of view, EpCAM is also highly expressed in premalignant hepatic lesions and could, therefore, be helpful to improve early detection of HCC. Interestingly, a subpopulation of EpCAM+ HCCs is also positive for CD133.

CD133 (Prominin 1) is a 5-transmembrane domain glycoprotein. High expression of CD133 has been described in CSCs from a variety of cancers including brain, prostate, pancreas and colon. After initial demonstration of CSC properties in HCC by Suetsugu et al., several studies confirmed the enrichment of stemness properties in CD133+ cells including a strong proliferative as well as differentiating capacity and a high tumorigenic potential [53, 70, 76–88]. Sasaki et al. further showed that cytoplasmatic expression of CD133 was associated with elevated AFP serum levels, higher histological grades and increased malignant portal vein invasion [70]. CD133 expression also correlated with advanced stages of disease, early recurrence and high chemo- as well as radio-resistance. Recent studies have revealed different molecular pathways involved in chemo- and radio-resistance of CD133+ cells including an activation of AKT/PKB signaling [61], IL6/STAT3 [62], an overexpression of ABC transporters [89] as well as reduced levels of reactive oxygen species [81]. Given the body of literature demonstrating the enrichment of putative CSCs by CD133, it is not surprising that different studies addressed the clinical importance of targeting cells with high levels of CD133 in HCC. Smith et al. showed that effective growth inhibition in HCC cell lines can be achieved targeting CD133 with an anti-CD133 antibody conjugated to monomethyl-auristatin-F, a potent cytotoxic drug [83]. Another study showed the inhibitory effect of transcription factor Ikaros on tumorigenic and self-renewal properties of CD133+ CSCs [76]. Herein, the inhibitory mechanism was conducted through direct binding of Ikaros to CD133 P1 promoter. Other studies suggest that the use of oncolytic viruses in HCC might specifically target CD133+ CSCs.

CD90 (Thy-1) is a glycosylphosphatidylinositol-anchored conserved surface marker widely expressed on different cell types such as T-cells, fibroblasts, neurons and endothelial cells [90]. Yang et al. identified CD90 as a potential CSCs marker in HCC after exclusion of hematopoietic cells by CD45 expression [54, 91]. Detection of CD90+/CD45− cells were observed in all investigated HCC cell lines and also in 31 out of 34 blood samples from HCC patients suggesting the presence of circulating CSCs. Since CD90+/CD45− cells were absent in blood samples of controls with normal liver function or liver cirrhosis, CD90 expression might be of diagnostic significance [54, 91].

CD44, is a cell surface glycoprotein acting as a receptor of hyaluronate and is often used in combination with other CSC markers such as CD133 and CD90 to improve identification of hepatic CSCs [54, 89, 92]. Functionally, CD44 is important for cell adhesion and migration. Co-expressing CD133+/CD44+ and CD90+/CD44+ cells had a more aggressive phenotype than CD90+ and CD133+ cells alone and effectively induced lung metastasis in immunocompromised mice [54, 89, 92]. Therefore, CD44 seems to play a key role in the development of distant metastases, which has a dramatic effect on the overall survival of HCC patients. Furthermore, therapy resistance is also closely linked with a high CD44 expression: After thermal ablation of liver cancer lesions in immunocompromised mice, CD44+ but not CD90+ cells were detected in the margin of the ablation and are, thus, possibly responsible for recurrence of cancer growth [93]. Evaluation of the therapeutic potential of targeting CD44 in HCC using neutralizing antibodies confirmed an anti-tumorigenic effect in vitro and in vivo [54]. Consistently, treatment of the HCC cell lines with the antibody induced apoptosis in a concentration-dependent manner, while in vivo administration of anti-CD44 antibodies in immunocompromised, tumor-bearing mice prevented liver tumor formation as well as lung metastasis.

CD24, is a mucin-like cell surface glycoprotein, also often co-expressed with CD133 or EpCAM and highly expressed in putative stem/progenitor cells [94]. The significance of this marker for a CSC phenotype has been evaluated is a variety of human cancers including liver cancer [95]. In HCC, functional studies revealed that CD24+ hepatospheres were larger in size than those induced by CD24− cells. Further, only few CD24+ cells were capable to initiate tumor development in immunodeficient mice [55, 73]. Furthermore, Yang et al. observed that CD24 was overexpressed in highly metastatic HCC cell lines as well as in tumor tissues of HCC patients with recurrent disease. CD24 overexpression is also associated with a poor outcome after surgery, in particular in patients with normal AFP, early stage and well-differentiated HCCs [96]. Additionally, CD24 expression seems to play an important role in maintaining (cancer-) stem cell features by regulating self-renewal and tumor initiation through STAT3-mediated NANOG regulation [73]. Interestingly, adjuvant transcatheter arterial chemoembolization (TACE) after surgery effectively reduced the rate of early recurrence in CD24+ HCC patients, while remained ineffective in CD24− HCC patients [96]. Therefore, evaluation of CD24 expression might not only be a promising prognostic marker but also helpful to predict response to treatment and guide therapeutic strategies.

CD13, Aminopeptidase N, is a membranous glycoprotein, which is mostly expressed during the G1/G0 phase of the cell cycle and seems to play a critical role for the development of relapse in HCC [97]. Haraguchi et al. identified CD13 as a functional membrane marker for dormant liver CSCs [98]. Immunohistochemical analysis showed that CD13+ cells survived TACE and were enriched near the fibrous capsule after treatment where recurrence of HCC is a frequent event. Components of the capsule could build a protective niche for CD13+ cells. Mechanistically, CD13+ cells possessed high resistance against ROS-induced DNA damage after chemo- or radiation-induced stress and were protected from apoptosis [98]. Further, administration of CD13-neutralizing antibodies or the protease inhibitor ubenimex significantly decreased self-renewal and tumor initiating ability of CD13+ CSCs [98].

OV6 marks putative hepatic progenitor cells located in the periportal region [52]. OV6+ cells have the ability to differentiate into hepatocytes or cholangiocytes. Yang et al. demonstrated that OV6+ HCC cells display higher tumorigenic and chemoresistant potential than OV6− cells [99]. Interestingly, OV6+ cells also co-expressed CD133+ suggesting that OV6 can also serve as a potential CSC marker. In vitro and in vivo studies further revealed that OV6+ tumor cells possessed stronger metastatic properties and were highly invasive. Importantly, high frequency of OV6+ cells was associated with a poor prognosis of HCC patients.

Side population approach (Hoechst-33342-dye staining), originally established in 1996 by Goodell et al. to isolate hematopoietic stem cells, is a widely used functional assay to identify stem cells as well as CSCs from different tissues [100]. Cells are sorted by flow-cytometry after Hoechst-33342 vital dye staining. A distinct population of cells, the so-called side population, which actively effluxes the dye due to high activity of ABC membrane transporters, can be discriminated by this approach. Among the different substrates are also several chemotherapeutic compounds. Therefore, the side population approach can be used as a surrogate characteristic for chemoresistance [15, 101]. Haraguchi et al. were the first describing CSC features in the side population of liver cancer cells in 2006 [102]. Since then, several studies confirmed enrichment of stemness genes, self-renewal and tumorigenic potential as well as metastatic capacities in SP cells [15, 101]. Global transcriptomic analysis of SP cells even revealed a common SP-gene expression signature that was closely associated with the clinical outcome of HCC patients [45].

In conclusion, several CSC markers have been extensively studied in the context of HCC. While some of the markers might have a potential in identifying patients at risk for early tumor recurrence or metastases and help to select individual therapeutic strategies, their detailed role as prognostic and/or predictive biomarkers remains controversial [82, 103, 104]. Furthermore, results from the above mentioned studies and lack of overlap between the different markers clearly indicate that not a single marker might be sufficient to identify the heterogeneous population of CSCs in HCC. In support of this, Yamashita et al. recently demonstrated that EpCAM and

CD90 are independently expressed in liver cancer [105]. While EpCAM+ cells displayed properties of epithelial cells and its expression was associated with poorly differentiated morphology as well as high serum AFP, CD90+ cells had features of vascular endothelial cells and were correlated with a high incidence of distant organ metastasis. Thus, assays based on functional properties or, even better, a combination of different functional and antigenic approaches might be more suitable for reliable identification of stem-like cells in HCC.

Cancer Stem Cell Regulation, Targeting and Mechanisms of Chemoresistance

Over the last decade, a more detailed understanding of the molecular events that govern tumor progression and dissemination of cancer has led to the development of targeted treatments that aim to interfere with specific, cancer-related signaling pathways [106]. Although promising novel therapies and molecular targets are currently under evaluation for liver cancer, the only approved systemic therapy for patients with advanced HCC remains sorafenib, with mean survival benefit of only 3 months [106–109]. Recent data have demonstrated survival benefits of regorafenib in patients that progressed after sorafenib [110]. Sorafenib is an oral multityrosinekinase-inhibitor which inhibits multiple cell surface and downstream kinases involved in tumor progression. Important signaling pathways affected by the treatment are RAS/RAF, VEGFR and PDGFR as well as c-Kit [111, 112]. Results from the clinical trials indicate that not all of the HCC patients treated with sorafenib show a survival benefit. This observation addresses an important question in HCC biology namely, the mechanisms of chemoresistance leading to treatment failure. Since drug resistance, relapse formation and metastatic spread are fundamental properties of CSCs, their importance for tumor biology, in particular for multi-resistant cancers such as HCC, are increasingly recognized [1]. As outlined in the above sections, many studies have tried to address clinical relevance of CSCs in HCC [8, 23, 107]. Some of the studies indicate that CSCs are enriched by classical chemotherapy and, thus, selective targeting of rapidly proliferating tumor cells might lead to reduction of the gross tumor mass, without affecting the cancer-sustaining CSCs [55]. These studies also indicate that CSCs might be induced, maintained and regulated by different molecular mechanisms than their more differentiated progeny. These stemness-associated signaling pathways are responsible for the maintenance of tumorigenic and metastatic properties as well as chemoresistance [113]. Therefore, the selective targeting of these pathways is one of the biggest challenges in the pursue to eradicate CSCs in HCC [55]. We describe below the most relevant signaling pathways that have been identified to be of relevance for (cancer-) stemness in the context of therapeutic approaches (Fig. 3).

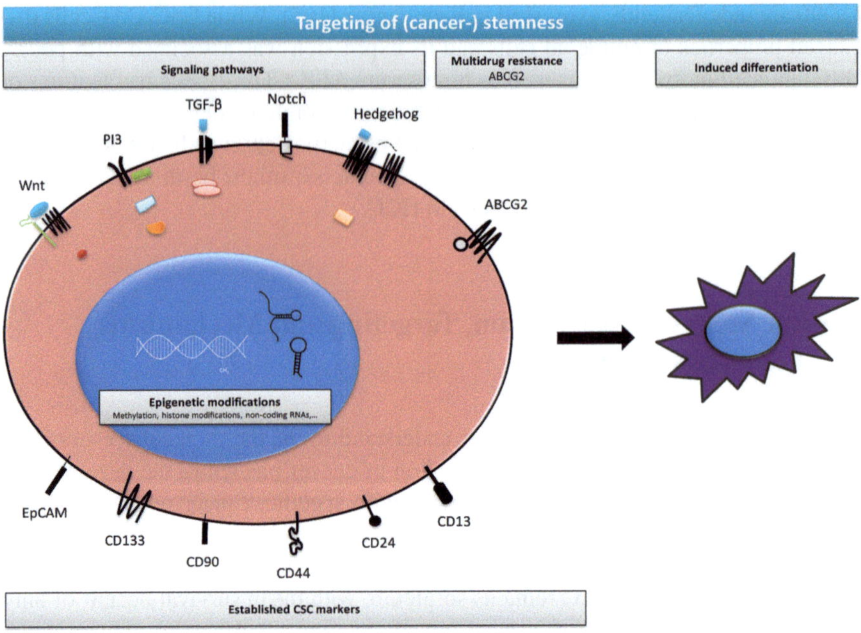

Fig. 3 Specific targeting of CSCs. CSCs are exclusively responsible for tumor initiation and progression. By definition, CSCs show a high resistance to chemotherapeutic compounds. Development of novel therapies specifically directed towards CSCs seem a promising therapeutic strategy in HCC. Therefore, the identification and targeting of stemness-related signaling pathways (WNT/β-catenin, TGF-β, PI3/AKT/mTOR, Notch, Hedgehog), CSC cell surface markers (EpCAM, CD133, CD90, CD44, CD24, CD13.), inhibition of multidrug resistance transporters (ABCG2) as well as epigenetic modifications (methylation, histone modifications, non-coding RNAs) seem promising. Another potential approach could also be the induction of differentiation in the stem-like cancer cells

Targeting Stemness-Related Signaling Pathways

Liver CSCs are likely to be dependent on a variety of mechanisms that support the stem-like phenotype of the cells by promoting self-renewal and pluripotency. Different signaling pathways such as WNT/β-catenin, TGF-β, PI3/AKT/mTOR, MET, Notch, Hedgehog, MYC, P53, among others, are known to play critical roles in the regulation and maintenance of stemness features under physiological conditions in the liver [114, 115]. The notion that many of these pathways are frequently re-activated and deregulation in cancer suggests that their induction plays a critical role in the formation of liver CSCs [22]. Therefore, specific targeting of these pathways or key components might be promising therapeutic approaches to eradicate CSCs and potentially avoid therapy resistance.

Wnt/β-catenin is an evolutionary conserved signaling pathway which plays an important role in many biological processes such as development, differentiation and cellular homeostasis [68]. In cancer, deregulation of this pathway is also frequently observed [116]. Compelling evidences indicate that activation of the Wnt/β--catenin signaling is crucial for driving hepatocarcinogenesis, particularly for the maintenance of a putative CSC compartment [115, 117]. In support of this notion, many of the identified CSC markers such as CD44, CD24, EpCAM, are also found to be Wnt target genes [118]. Consistently, several studies also demonstrated that Wnt activation can significantly increase EpCAM+ CSC populations and potentiate their self-renewal capacity [75, 116, 119]. Furthermore, Wnt/β-catenin induces the expression of certain microRNAs (e.g. microRNA-181) resulting in enhanced stemness features of EpCAM+ CSC populations [120, 121]. A study by Mokkapati et al. also emphasizes the crucial role of Wnt/β-catenin for tumor initiation in HCC [122]. The authors identified a unique population of progenitor cells in fetal livers marked by the expression of the cited1-CreERTM-GFP transgene. Upon stabilization of β-catenin in these cells, over 90% of transgenic mice by 26 weeks of age developed intrahepatic and metastatic liver tumors. Moreover, the expression of hepatic stem/progenitor cell markers as well as activation of the RAS/RAF/MAPK and PI3K/AKT/mTOR pathways were also observed. However, although targeting of Wnt/β--catenin signaling is overall challenging, new discoveries introducing a new class of potential inhibitors might have profound effects for hepatic CSC eradication [123].

TGF-β signaling is involved in various cellular functions such as cell growth, differentiation and apoptosis [124]. In healthy tissue, TGF-β has protective effects by controlling the cell cycle, inducing apoptosis and regulating autophagy [125]. During hepatocarcinogenesis, this tumor suppressing effect of TGF-β is disrupted at later stages, which promotes metastatic and invasive properties as well as chemoresistance and CSC maintenance [87, 126, 127]. Wu et al. reported an association of TGF-β with CSC formation during hepatocarcinogenesis [127]. The authors showed that TGF-β facilitated malignant transformation of liver progenitor cells into hepatic CSCs via hyperactivation of Akt. Another study demonstrated that HCC cells with activation of the TGF-β pathway display a mesenchymal-like phenotype and a high expression of the CSC marker CD44. These cells were also highly resistant to sorafenib-induced cell death. Conversely, epithelial-like cells expressing CSC markers EpCAM and CD133 showed high sensitivity to the treatment after inhibition of CD44. From these results the authors conclude that CD44 plays a key role in protecting the cells from sorafenib-induced apoptosis and that its expression as well as acquisition of a mesenchymal phenotype is mediated by TGF-β signaling [128]. Notably, the response to sorafenib was also inversely correlated to CD133 expression as well as the JNK pathway activity [77]. However, targeting TGF-β in CSCs is still very hard to achieve and might induce differential effects in HCC and other resident liver cells. Nevertheless, targeting strategies to specifically inhibit TGF-β in tumor cells by siRNA as well as blocking of ligand-receptor interactions by monoclonal antibodies or small molecule inhibitors are underway [129].

PI3/AKT/mTOR An increasing number of studies confirms the relevance of the PI3/AKT/mTOR pathway for a diverse range of physiological and pathological conditions such as proliferation, differentiation, survival and tumorigenesis [63]. Disruption of this signaling pathway in normal cells can result in malignant transformation [63]. Intriguingly, activation of PI3/AKT/mTOR in the liver also promotes the development of HCCs with less differentiated phenotypes and poor prognosis [130]. Recently, Su et al. confirmed the crucial role of PTEN/AKT/mTOR in particular for tumor recurrence and prognosis of HCC patients [64]. The authors also showed a significant relationship between liver CSCs and components of this pathway. Resulting from these investigations they propose a combination of PTEN with CD133 or EpCAM as a potential prognostic tool. In line with this, Ma et al. demonstrated an association between CD133+ putative CSCs and chemoresistance by activation of the AKT/PKB as well as BCL-2 pro-survival signaling [61]. Furthermore, the interaction between AKT and HIF-1α might confer to hypoxia-mediated chemoresistance of liver CSCs [131]. Under hypoxic conditions, AKT and HIF-1 were up-regulated and formed an autocrine signaling loop with PDGF-β, which resulted in resistance to cisplatin treatment. Moreover, the ability of CD133+ CSCs to evade irradiation could be attributed to activation of the MAPK/PI3K pathway [81]. As PI3/AKT/mTOR might be one of the central players in HCC, blocking this pathway is attractive strategy to treat CSCs and overcome resistance in HCC.

Notch signaling is evolutionarily highly conserved and plays an important role in many developmental processes such as differentiation, cell fate decision, proliferation, apoptosis, cell adhesion and regulation of stem/progenitor states [132]. Despite recent evidence for Notch activation in some solid tumors, the exact role of this pathway for HCC as well as CSCs still remains controversial [133, 134]. Viatour et al. showed that activation of Notch signaling in HCC might even act as a potent tumor suppressor [135]. Although activation of this pathway was not sufficient to prevent initiation of the tumor, tumor growth was significantly reduced. In contrast, other studies suggest that Notch signaling might even promote hepatocarcinogenesis in a genetically-modified mouse model [132]. The authors further showed that activation of this pathway is observed in around one third of human HCC patients. Further, inhibition of the Notch pathway with specific y-secretase inhibitors might potentially inhibit CSC self-renewal and tumor growth [136]. Notably, the described opposing effects of the Notch pathway on tumor initiation and progression might be due to different disease etiologies, complex micro-environmental influences as well as many other factors. Despite the undisputed importance for liver cancer, dissection and characterization of its regulatory effects and downstream targets in HCC are needed before a putative therapeutic application is warranted.

Hedgehog (Hh) signaling is essential for progenitor cell fate decisions, proliferation, apoptosis, migration and differentiation [137, 138]. Important effects mediated by activation of the Hh signaling in liver tissue are expansion of progenitor cells during liver regeneration, accumulation of inflammatory cells and vascular remodeling [137, 139, 140]. Growing evidence further indicates that Hh signaling is frequently activated in many liver cancers [141, 142]. Accumulating evidence also shows that upregulation of *Shh* might contribute to malignant transformation of hepatocytes [143]. In addition, Hh signaling might be closely interacting with other cancer related pathways such as Wnt/β-catenin and c-Myc during hepatocarcinogenesis [144, 145]. Consistently, specific inhibition of SMO (major signal transducer of Shh pathway) with KAAD-cyclopamine caused decreased expression of c-Myc, one of the key oncogenic factors in hepatocarcinogenesis [142, 145]. Targeted therapy of Hh signaling by KAAD-cyclopamine, a known SMO antagonist, or Hh neutralizing antibodies led to activation of apoptosis and considerable tumor regression in HCC.

Targeting Drug Resistance: ABCG2 Transporter

The adenosine triphosphate (ATP)-binding cassette G2 (ABCG2) is of great importance in HCC biology, in particular for the characterization of putative scarce CSCs within the tumor mass [55, 146]. As mentioned before, the ability of ABCG2 transporter to actively efflux Hoechst-33342-dye can be utilized for the detection of putative CSCs. Besides effluxing Hoechst-33342-dye, this protein operates as a xenobiotic transporter and might play an important role in multi-drug resistance to chemotherapeutic agents [15]. A study by Wang et al. showed a close association between the stem cell transcriptional factor OCT4 and the expression of ABCG2 transporter [146]. The results of this study implied that inhibition of the OCT4-TCL1-AKT pathway might influence cell survival and drug sensitivity in CSCs by affecting the regulation of the ABCG2 transporter. Jia et al. later confirmed the association between OCT4 and ABCG2 in liver CSCs [78]. Both genes were highly expressed in enriched CD90+ CD133+ liver CSCs and resembled drug resistance of these cells. Furthermore, less differentiated HCC cell lines show high level of ABCG2 expression and high functional activity of the transporter [147]. The available data, therefore, suggest that high expression and activity of the ABCG2 transporter can promote chemoresistant properties of CSCs. Therefore, the ABCG2 transporter might be an interesting molecular target.

Differentiation Therapy

Driving differentiation of cancer cells, in particular CSCs, is an emerging new therapeutic approach. The approach is based on the hypothesis that quiescent CSCs can be forced to differentiate and form less tumorigenic progeny that lack self-renewing and invasive properties [55]. Loss of stem-like characteristics might also render them more susceptible to conventional therapy. Several factors have been found to play a role in the differentiation of hepatic progenitor cells into mature hepatocytes. Among them are well known molecules such as Oncostatin M (OSM) and Hepatocyte nuclear factor-4α (HNF4α) [148]. Consistently, forced activation of these molecules and related signaling pathways lead to differentiation and loss of stem-like properties in the hepatic CSC compartment [149]. These interesting findings might indicate that the combination of forced differentiation with traditional therapeutic approaches is promising to improve treatment of HCC.

Epigenetic Modifications and CSC Therapy

The current concept emphasizes that cancer arises as the consequence of adverse genetic and epigenetic events [150]. Epigenetic alterations cause changes in the expression of genes and proteins without changing the DNA sequence. Epigenetic changes are frequently found during tumor initiation and progression of many cancers [147, 151]. Not surprising, epigenetic modifications also play a key role in hepatocarcinogenesis. Global hypomethylation and promoter hypermethylation are supposed to be among the most common and early events during hepatocarcinogenesis [152]. Wang et al. demonstrated that epigenetic modifications induce the expression of pluripotency-associated genes such as *OCT4, c-MYC, KLF4, SOX2*, particularly *NANOG* in cancer cells [153]. Results of the study support the concept of an epigenetic oncogenic reprogramming that is critical for CSC development. Confirming this finding, DNA methylation was identified as a key epigenetic regulator for maintenance of CSC properties in HCC [45]. The study utilized the DNA methyltransferases inhibitor (DNMT1-inhibitor) zebularine to epigenetically modify putative CSCs. Epigenetic modification caused a dramatic enrichment of highly tumorigenic CSCs within the SP fraction, thereby, leading to an improved discrimination. The importance of demethylation for the CSC biology was confirmed in a study by You et al. demonstrating that TGF-β regulates CD133 expression through promotor demethylation by inhibiting DNMT1 and DNMT3B [87]. Evaluation of compounds interfering with the epigenome of HCC cells might, therefore, be a promising treatment strategy. Several epigenetic modifying agents are currently under clinical evaluation. Besides demethylating compounds such as 5-azacytidine, DNMT1-inhibitor zebularine, HDAC inhibitors such as resminostat showed promising results in phase II clinical trials on HCC [154].

MicroRNAs (miRNAs) are small non-coding RNAs involved in post-transcriptional regulation of many protein coding genes. Over the recent years, miRNAs have emerged to important molecules in tumor therapy [57, 155]. Thus, modulating the expression of miRNAs might also be a potentially useful tool for specific targeting of CSCs. Many studies have reported that deregulation of several miRNAs is closely linked with tumor development and seeding of metastases in HCC [58, 59]. Meng et al. showed that specific transcriptional factors are regulating levels of miRNAs with crucial importance for the induction of chemoresistance of CSCs. The study showed that IL-6 regulates the expression of let-7 and miR-181, thereby, leading to activation of the pro-metastatic transcriptional factor Twist. Concomitant to increased levels of these miRNAs, tumor cells demonstrated higher chemoresistance against sorafenib and doxorubicin [60]. Consistently, miR-181 might also effectively diminish EpCAM+ liver CSCs [120]. Further, high expression of miR-491 effectively attenuated CSC-like properties and EMT features in HCC cell lines [156].

Another important group of non-coding RNAs, also known as long non-coding RNAs (lncRNAs), was recently recognized as an important player in the development and progression of cancer [72]. By definition, lncRNAs are RNA transcripts consisting of more than 200 nucleotides and without protein coding function [157]. They are known to be involved in different regulatory processes ranging from transcriptional and post-transcriptional regulation to epigenetic modifications. In this context, they might affect a diverse range of signaling pathways with a crucial role in hepatocarcinogenesis. Moreover, they may modulate cell response to anticancer agents and lead to failure of systemic therapies [71]. There are several studies addressing the association between lncRNAs and CSC properties in liver cancer. In the study of Wang et al., the authors reported that lnc-DILC (lncRNA downregulated in liver cancer stem cells) dramatically effects CSC self-renewal [158]. lnc-DILC suppressed CSC expansion by affecting IL-6 as well as STAT3 signaling. Moreover, the data suggest that lnc-DILC operates as an essential mediator between NF-κB activation and IL-6 expression in CSCs, which confirms the known interplay between hepatic inflammation and CSC induction. CUDR (long noncoding RNA cancer upregulated drug resistant) is another lncRNA overexpressed in many tumors. Gui et al. demonstrated the impact of CUDR on liver CSCs through regulating the cascade of CUDR-HULC(highly upregulated in liver cancer)/CUDR-β-catenin signaling. This cascade provides a potentially novel regulatory link between oncogenic function of lncRNA and the epigenetic modification of CSCs [69]. Several other lncRNAs have been found to contribute to the pathogenesis and progression of HCC such as MALAT-1, which is involved in mRNA splicing and cell cycle regulation [159, 160], as well as HOTAIR, which modulates epigenetic repression of PCR2 target genes [65, 161]. Based on these recent findings in this field, lncRNAs might become attractive novel therapeutic tools for HCC.

Summary and Future Challenges for Cancer Stem Cell Research in HCC

CSCs are primarily responsible for cancer initiation, local recurrence, seeding of metastasis as well as therapy resistance. Current evidence further suggests that recently applied cancer therapies for liver cancer predominantly target rapidly dividing, well differentiated cells while leaving the CSCs unharmed. This observation may also partly explain the disappointing results of ongoing clinical phase II-III clinical trials in HCC [162]. Consequently, targeting CSCs should become the primary focus of translational efforts and might be helpful to overcome resistance in HCC. In support of this, a recent study confirms that acquired resistance to sorafenib treatment is mainly driven by aberrant CSCs that display activation of IGF and FGF signaling pathways [163]. Since these investigations suggest that inhibition of CSC pathways would confer a treatment benefit for HCC patients, it is important to emphasize the necessity to explore the susceptibility of CSC to existing therapies in combination with the disruption of key stemness pathways resembling self-renewal, pluripotency, radio-chemoresistance as well as neo-angiogenesis. Other novel and potentially important directions for effective therapy may include disruption of the tumor niche which is essential for CSC homeostasis as well as depletion of CSCs.

Despite a controversial relevance in predicting prognosis of HCC, targeting of CSC specific surface markers, such as CD133, CD90, CD13, EpCAM and CD44, or pluripotency factors may also be a promising approach to specifically target hepatic CSCs [164]. However, these approaches require great caution due to context-dependence and redundancy in adult tissue stem cells and the CSCs. Therefore, great efforts should be made to improve pre-clinical models that closely mimic the human disease. In this context, the development and propagation of patient-derived tumor cells as well as mouse models that allow to studying the impact of the diseased microenvironment and the interaction of tumor, stromal and immune cells will become particularly important [66, 67].

Collectively, compelling evidence over the recent years suggests a hierarchic organization of liver cancer. Results of recent studies strongly emphasize the potential of specific targeting the CSC to complement existing therapies and overcome drug resistance. Therefore, evaluation of novel therapeutic approaches that combine chemotherapeutic compounds with CSC-directed therapies seems most promising.

Acknowledgement J.U.M. is supported by grants from the German Research Foundation (MA 4443/2-2), the German Cancer Aid (DKH 110989) and the Volkswagen Foundation (Lichtenberg program). C.C. is supported by a fellowship grant from the Transmed Program of the Universitätsmedizin Mainz.

Disclosure Nothing to disclose.

References

1. Marquardt JU, Factor VM, Thorgeirsson SS. Epigenetic regulation of cancer stem cells in liver cancer: current concepts and clinical implications. J Hepatol. 2010;53:568–77.
2. Bergsagel DE, Valeriote FA. Growth characteristics of a mouse plasma cell tumor. Cancer Res. 1968;28:2187–96.
3. Hamburger AW, Salmon SE. Primary bioassay of human tumor stem cells. Science. 1977;197:461–3.
4. Heppner GH. Tumor heterogeneity. Cancer Res. 1984;44:2259–65.
5. Reya T, Morrison SJ, Clarke MF, Weissman IL. Stem cells, cancer, and cancer stem cells. Nature. 2001;414:105–11.
6. Southam CM, Brunschwig A. Quantitative studies of autotransplantation of human cancer – preliminary report. Cancer. 1961;14:971.
7. Visvader JE, Lindeman GJ. Cancer stem cells in solid tumours: accumulating evidence and unresolved questions. Nat Rev Cancer. 2008;8:755–68.
8. Jordan CT, Guzman ML, Noble M. Cancer stem cells. N Engl J Med. 2006;355:1253–61.
9. Dean M, Fojo T, Bates S. Tumour stem cells and drug resistance. Nat Rev Cancer. 2005;5:275–84.
10. Llovet JM, Ricci S, Mazzaferro V, Hilgard P, Gane E, Blanc JF, et al. Sorafenib in advanced hepatocellular carcinoma. N Engl J Med. 2008;359:378–90.
11. Mueller MT, Hermann PC, Witthauer J, Rubio-Viqueira B, Leicht SF, Huber S, et al. Combined targeted treatment to eliminate tumorigenic cancer stem cells in human pancreatic cancer. Gastroenterology. 2009;137:1102–13.

12. Trumpp A, Wiestler OD. Mechanisms of disease: cancer stem cells--targeting the evil twin. Nat Clin Pract Oncol. 2008;5:337–47.
13. Visvader JE, Lindeman GJ. Cancer stem cells: current status and evolving complexities. Cell Stem Cell. 2012;10:717–28.
14. Duncan AW, Dorrell C, Grompe M. Stem cells and liver regeneration. Gastroenterology. 2009;137:466–81.
15. Chiba T, Kita K, Zheng YW, Yokosuka O, Saisho H, Iwama A, et al. Side population purified from hepatocellular carcinoma cells harbors cancer stem cell-like properties. Hepatology. 2006;44:240–51.
16. Hermann PC, Huber SL, Herrler T, Aicher A, Ellwart JW, Guba M, et al. Distinct populations of cancer stem cells determine tumor growth and metastatic activity in human pancreatic cancer. Cell Stem Cell. 2007;1:313–23.
17. Ma S, Chan KW, Hu L, Lee TK, Wo JY, Ng IO, et al. Identification and characterization of tumorigenic liver cancer stem/progenitor cells. Gastroenterology. 2007;132:2542–56.
18. Nowell PC. Clonal evolution of tumor-cell populations. Science. 1976;194:23–8.
19. Clarke MF, Dick JE, Dirks PB, Eaves CJ, Jamieson CH, Jones DL, et al. Cancer stem cells--perspectives on current status and future directions: AACR workshop on cancer stem cells. Cancer Res. 2006;66:9339–44.
20. Merlo LM, Maley CC. The role of genetic diversity in cancer. J Clin Invest. 2010;120:401–3.
21. Kakarala M, Wicha MS. Implications of the cancer stem-cell hypothesis for breast cancer prevention and therapy. J Clin Oncol. 2008;26:2813–20.
22. Marquardt JU, Thorgeirsson SS. Stem cells in hepatocarcinogenesis: evidence from genomic data. Semin Liver Dis. 2010;30:26–34.
23. Llovet JM, Bruix J. Molecular targeted therapies in hepatocellular carcinoma. Hepatology. 2008;48:1312–27.
24. Durnez A, Verslype C, Nevens F, Fevery J, Aerts R, Pirenne J, et al. The clinicopathological and prognostic relevance of cytokeratin 7 and 19 expression in hepatocellular carcinoma. A possible progenitor cell origin. Histopathology. 2006;49:138–51.
25. Libbrecht L, Desmet V, Van DB, Roskams T. The immunohistochemical phenotype of dysplastic foci in human liver: correlation with putative progenitor cells. J Hepatol. 2000;33:76–84.
26. He G, Dhar D, Nakagawa H, Font-Burgada J, Ogata H, Jiang Y, et al. Identification of liver cancer progenitors whose malignant progression depends on autocrine IL-6 signaling. Cell. 2013;155:384–96.
27. Lee JS. A novel prognostic subtype of human hepatocellular carcinoma derived from hepatic progenitor cells. Nat Med. 2006;12:410–6.
28. Woo HG, Wang XW, Budhu A, Kim YH, Kwon SM, Tang ZY, et al. Association of TP53 mutations with stem cell-like gene expression and survival of patients with hepatocellular carcinoma. Gastroenterology. 2011;140:1063–70.
29. Yamashita T, Ji J, Budhu A, Forgues M, Yang W, Wang HY, et al. EpCAM-positive hepatocellular carcinoma cells are tumor-initiating cells with stem/progenitor cell features. Gastroenterology. 2009;136:1012–24.
30. Mu X, Espanol-Suner R, Mederacke I, Affo S, Manco R, Sempoux C, et al. Hepatocellular carcinoma originates from hepatocytes and not from the progenitor/biliary compartment. J Clin Invest. 2015;125:3891–903.
31. Font-Burgada J, Shalapour S, Ramaswamy S, Hsueh B, Rossell D, Umemura A, et al. Hybrid periportal hepatocytes regenerate the injured liver without giving rise to cancer. Cell. 2015;162:766–79.
32. Fan B, Malato Y, Calvisi DF, Naqvi S, Razumilava N, Ribback S, et al. Cholangiocarcinomas can originate from hepatocytes in mice. J Clin Invest. 2012;122:2911–5.
33. Holczbauer A, Factor VM, Andersen JB, Marquardt JU, Kleiner D, Raggi C, et al. Modeling pathogenesis of primary liver cancer in lineage-specific mouse cell types. Gastroenterology. 2013;145:221–31.

34. Akita H, Marquardt JU, Durkin ME, Kitade M, Seo D, Conner EA, et al. MYC activates stem-like cell potential in hepatocarcinoma by a p53-dependent mechanism. Cancer Res. 2014;74:5903–13.
35. Marquardt JU, Thorgeirsson SS. Sall4 in "stemness"-driven hepatocarcinogenesis. N Engl J Med. 2013;368:2316–8.
36. Schoenhals M, Kassambara A, De VJ, Hose D, Moreaux J, Klein B. Embryonic stem cell markers expression in cancers. Biochem Biophys Res Commun. 2009;383:157–62.
37. Oikawa T, Kamiya A, Zeniya M, Chikada H, Hyuck AD, Yamazaki Y, et al. Sal-like protein 4 (SALL4), a stem cell biomarker in liver cancers. Hepatology. 2013;57:1469–83.
38. Yong KJ, Gao C, Lim JS, Yan B, Yang H, Dimitrov T, et al. Oncofetal gene SALL4 in aggressive hepatocellular carcinoma. N Engl J Med. 2013;368:2266–76.
39. Luedde T, Schwabe RF. NF-kappaB in the liver--linking injury, fibrosis and hepatocellular carcinoma. Nat Rev Gastroenterol Hepatol. 2011;8:108–18.
40. Zhao W, Wang L, Han H, Jin K, Lin N, Guo T, et al. 1B50-1, a mAb raised against recurrent tumor cells, targets liver tumor-initiating cells by binding to the calcium channel alpha2delta1 subunit. Cancer Cell. 2013;23:541–56.
41. Hoshida Y, Villanueva A, Kobayashi M, Peix J, Chiang DY, Camargo A, et al. Gene expression in fixed tissues and outcome in hepatocellular carcinoma. N Engl J Med. 2008;359:1995–2004.
42. Maeda S, Hikiba Y, Sakamoto K, Nakagawa H, Hirata Y, Hayakawa Y, et al. Ikappa B kinasebeta/nuclear factor-kappaB activation controls the development of liver metastasis by way of interleukin-6 expression. Hepatology. 2009;50:1851–60.
43. Elsharkawy AM, Mann DA. Nuclear factor-kappaB and the hepatic inflammation-fibrosis-cancer axis. Hepatology. 2007;46:590–7.
44. Feng GS. Conflicting roles of molecules in hepatocarcinogenesis: paradigm or paradox. Cancer Cell. 2012;21:150–4.
45. Marquardt JU, Raggi C, Andersen JB, Seo D, Avital I, Geller D, et al. Human hepatic cancer stem cells are characterized by common stemness traits and diverse oncogenic pathways. Hepatology. 2011;54:1031–42.
46. Karin M. Nuclear factor-kappaB in cancer development and progression. Nature. 2006;441:431–6.
47. Marquardt JU, Gomez-Quiroz L, Arreguin Camacho LO, Pinna F, Lee YH, Kitade M, et al. Curcumin effectively inhibits oncogenic NF-κB signaling and restrains stemness features in liver cancer. J Hepatol. 2015;63:661–9.
48. Govaere O, Wouters J, Petz M, Vandewynckel YP, Van den Eynde K, Van den Broeck A, et al. Laminin-332 sustains chemoresistance and quiescence as part of the human hepatic cancer stem cell niche. J Hepatol. 2016;64:609–17.
49. Plaks V, Kong N, Werb Z. The cancer stem cell niche: how essential is the niche in regulating stemness of tumor cells? Cell Stem Cell. 2015;16:225–38.
50. Marquardt JU, Nguyen-Tat M, Galle PR, Wörns MA. Surveillance of hepatocellular carcinoma and diagnostic algorithms in patients with liver cirrhosis. Visc Med. 2016;32:110–5.
51. Bialecki ES, Di Bisceglie AM. Diagnosis of hepatocellular carcinoma. HPB. 2005;7:26–34.
52. Romano M, De Francesco F, Pirozzi G, Gringeri E, Boetto R, Di Domenico M, et al. Expression of cancer stem cell biomarkers as a tool for a correct therapeutic approach to hepatocellular carcinoma. Oncoscience. 2015;2:443–56.
53. Ma S, Chan KW, Lee TK, Tang KH, Wo JY, Zheng BJ, et al. Aldehyde dehydrogenase discriminates the CD133 liver cancer stem cell populations. Mol Cancer Res. 2008;6:1146–53.
54. Yang ZF, Ho DW, Ng MN, Lau CK, Yu WC, Ngai P, et al. Significance of CD90+ cancer stem cells in human liver cancer. Cancer Cell. 2008;13:153–66.
55. Ji J, Wang XW. Clinical implications of cancer stem cell biology in hepatocellular carcinoma. Semin Oncol. 2012;39:461–72.
56. Yamashita T, Forgues M, Wang W, Kim JW, Ye Q, Jia H, et al. EpCAM and alpha-fetoprotein expression defines novel prognostic subtypes of hepatocellular carcinoma. Cancer Res. 2008;68:1451–61.

57. Callegari E, Gramantieri L, Domenicali M, D'Abundo L, Sabbioni S, Negrini M. MicroRNAs in liver cancer: a model for investigating pathogenesis and novel therapeutic approaches. Cell Death Differ. 2015;22:46–57.
58. Pang F, Zha R, Zhao Y, Wang Q, Chen D, Zhang Z, et al. MiR-525-3p enhances the migration and invasion of liver cancer cells by downregulating ZNF395. PLoS One. 2014;9:e90867.
59. Yao J, Liang L, Huang S, Ding J, Tan N, Zhao Y, et al. MicroRNA-30d promotes tumor invasion and metastasis by targeting Galphai2 in hepatocellular carcinoma. Hepatology. 2010;51:846–56.
60. Meng F, Glaser SS, Francis H, DeMorrow S, Han Y, Passarini JD, et al. Functional analysis of microRNAs in human hepatocellular cancer stem cells. J Cell Mol Med. 2012;16:160–73.
61. Ma S, Lee TK, Zheng BJ, Chan KW, Guan XY. CD133+ HCC cancer stem cells confer chemoresistance by preferential expression of the Akt/PKB survival pathway. Oncogene. 2008;27:1749–58.
62. Won C, Kim BH, Yi EH, Choi KJ, Kim EK, Jeong JM, et al. Signal transducer and activator of transcription 3-mediated CD133 up-regulation contributes to promotion of hepatocellular carcinoma. Hepatology. 2015;62:1160–73.
63. Polivka J Jr, Janku F. Molecular targets for cancer therapy in the PI3K/AKT/mTOR pathway. Pharmacol Ther. 2014;142:164–75.
64. Su R, Nan H, Guo H, Ruan Z, Jiang L, Song Y, et al. Associations of components of PTEN/AKT/mTOR pathway with cancer stem cell markers and prognostic value of these biomarkers in hepatocellular carcinoma. Hepatol Res. 2016;46:1380–91.
65. Tsai MC, Manor O, Wan Y, Mosammaparast N, Wang JK, Lan F, et al. Long noncoding RNA as modular scaffold of histone modification complexes. Science. 2010;329:689–93.
66. Sato T, Clevers H. SnapShot: growing organoids from stem cells. Cell. 2015;161:1700. e1701
67. Chen X, Calvisi DF. Hydrodynamic transfection for generation of novel mouse models for liver cancer research. Am J Pathol. 2014;184:912–23.
68. Logan CY, Nusse R. The Wnt signaling pathway in development and disease. Annu Rev Cell Dev Biol. 2004;20:781–810.
69. Gui X, Li H, Li T, Pu H, Lu D. Long noncoding RNA CUDR regulates HULC and beta-catenin to govern human liver stem cell malignant differentiation. Mol Ther. 2015;23:1843–53.
70. Sasaki A, Kamiyama T, Yokoo H, Nakanishi K, Kubota K, Haga H, et al. Cytoplasmic expression of CD133 is an important risk factor for overall survival in hepatocellular carcinoma. Oncol Rep. 2010;24:537–46.
71. Ghidini M, Braconi C. Non-coding RNAs in primary liver cancer. Front Med. 2015;2:36.
72. Huarte M, Rinn JL. Large non-coding RNAs: missing links in cancer? Hum Mol Genet. 2010;19:R152–61.
73. Lee TK, Castilho A, Cheung VC, Tang KH, Ma S, Ng IO. CD24(+) liver tumor-initiating cells drive self-renewal and tumor initiation through STAT3-mediated NANOG regulation. Cell Stem Cell. 2011;9:50–63.
74. Schmelzer E, Reid LM. EpCAM expression in normal, non-pathological tissues. Front Biosci. 2008;13:3096–100.
75. Yamashita T, Budhu A, Forgues M, Wang XW. Activation of hepatic stem cell marker EpCAM by Wnt-beta-catenin signaling in hepatocellular carcinoma. Cancer Res. 2007;67:10831–9.
76. Bach P, Abel T, Hoffmann C, Gal Z, Braun G, Voelker I, et al. Specific elimination of CD133+ tumor cells with targeted oncolytic measles virus. Cancer Res. 2013;73:865–74.
77. Hagiwara S, Kudo M, Nagai T, Inoue T, Ueshima K, Nishida N, et al. Activation of JNK and high expression level of CD133 predict a poor response to sorafenib in hepatocellular carcinoma. Br J Cancer. 2012;106:1997–2003.
78. Jia Q, Zhang X, Deng T, Gao J. Positive correlation of Oct4 and ABCG2 to chemotherapeutic resistance in CD90(+)CD133(+) liver cancer stem cells. Cell Reprogram. 2013;15:143–50.
79. Lin L, Amin R, Gallicano GI, Glasgow E, Jogunoori W, Jessup JM, et al. The STAT3 inhibitor NSC 74859 is effective in hepatocellular cancers with disrupted TGF-beta signaling. Oncogene. 2009;28:961–72.

80. Ma S, Tang KH, Chan YP, Lee TK, Kwan PS, Castilho A, et al. miR-130b Promotes CD133(+) liver tumor-initiating cell growth and self-renewal via tumor protein 53-induced nuclear protein 1. Cell Stem Cell. 2010;7:694–707.
81. Piao LS, Hur W, Kim TK, Hong SW, Kim SW, Choi JE, et al. CD133+ liver cancer stem cells modulate radioresistance in human hepatocellular carcinoma. Cancer Lett. 2012;315:129–37.
82. Salnikov AV, Kusumawidjaja G, Rausch V, Bruns H, Gross W, Khamidjanov A, et al. Cancer stem cell marker expression in hepatocellular carcinoma and liver metastases is not sufficient as single prognostic parameter. Cancer Lett. 2009;275:185–93.
83. Smith LM, Nesterova A, Ryan MC, Duniho S, Jonas M, Anderson M, et al. CD133/prominin-1 is a potential therapeutic target for antibody-drug conjugates in hepatocellular and gastric cancers. Br J Cancer. 2008;99:100–9.
84. Suetsugu A, Nagaki M, Aoki H, Motohashi T, Kunisada T, Moriwaki H. Characterization of CD133+ hepatocellular carcinoma cells as cancer stem/progenitor cells. Biochem Biophys Res Commun. 2006;351:820–4.
85. Tang KH, Ma S, Lee TK, Chan YP, Kwan PS, Tong CM, et al. CD133(+) liver tumor-initiating cells promote tumor angiogenesis, growth, and self-renewal through neurotensin/interleukin-8/CXCL1 signaling. Hepatology. 2012;55:807–20.
86. Yin S, Li J, Hu C, Chen X, Yao M, Yan M, et al. CD133 positive hepatocellular carcinoma cells possess high capacity for tumorigenicity. Int J Cancer. 2007;120:1444–50.
87. You H, Ding W, Rountree CB. Epigenetic regulation of cancer stem cell marker CD133 by transforming growth factor-beta. Hepatology. 2010;51:1635–44.
88. Zhu Z, Hao X, Yan M, Yao M, Ge C, Gu J, et al. Cancer stem/progenitor cells are highly enriched in CD133(+)CD44(+) population in hepatocellular carcinoma. Int J Cancer. 2009;26:2067–78.
89. Zhu Z, Hao X, Yan M, Yao M, Ge C, Gu J, et al. Cancer stem/progenitor cells are highly enriched in CD133+CD44+ population in hepatocellular carcinoma. Int J Cancer. 2010;126:2067–78.
90. Rege TA, Hagood JS. Thy-1 as a regulator of cell-cell and cell-matrix interactions in axon regeneration, apoptosis, adhesion, migration, cancer, and fibrosis. FASEB J. 2006;20:1045–54.
91. Yang ZF, Ngai P, Ho DW, Yu WC, Ng MN, Lau CK, et al. Identification of local and circulating cancer stem cells in human liver cancer. Hepatology. 2008;47:919–28.
92. Hou Y, Zou Q, Ge R, Shen F, Wang Y. The critical role of CD133(+)CD44(+/high) tumor cells in hematogenous metastasis of liver cancers. Cell Res. 2012;22:259–72.
93. Thompson SM, Callstrom MR, Butters KA, Sutor SL, Knudsen B, Grande JP, et al. Role for putative hepatocellular carcinoma stem cell subpopulations in biological response to incomplete thermal ablation: in vitro and in vivo pilot study. Cardiovasc Intervent Radiol. 2014;37:1343–51.
94. Shackleton M, Vaillant F, Simpson KJ, Stingl J, Smyth GK, Asselin-Labat ML, et al. Generation of a functional mammary gland from a single stem cell. Nature. 2006;439:84–8.
95. Burgos-Ojeda D, Wu R, McLean K, Chen YC, Talpaz M, Yoon E, et al. CD24+ ovarian cancer cells are enriched for cancer-initiating cells and dependent on JAK2 signaling for growth and metastasis. Mol Cancer Ther. 2015;14:1717–27.
96. Yang XR, Xu Y, Yu B, Zhou J, Li JC, Qiu SJ, et al. CD24 is a novel predictor for poor prognosis of hepatocellular carcinoma after surgery. Clin Cancer Res. 2009;15:5518–27.
97. Christ B, Stock P, Dollinger MM. CD13: Waving the flag for a novel cancer stem cell target. Hepatology. 2011;53:1388–90.
98. Haraguchi N, Ishii H, Mimori K, Tanaka F, Ohkuma M, Kim HM, et al. CD13 is a therapeutic target in human liver cancer stem cells. J Clin Invest. 2010;120:3326–39.
99. Yang W, Wang C, Lin Y, Liu Q, Yu LX, Tang L, et al. OV6(+) tumor-initiating cells contribute to tumor progression and invasion in human hepatocellular carcinoma. J Hepatol. 2012;57:613–20.
100. Goodell MA, Brose K, Paradis G, Conner AS, Mulligan RC. Isolation and functional properties of murine hematopoietic stem cells that are replicating in vivo. J Exp Med. 1996;183:1797–806.

101. Shi GM, Xu Y, Fan J, Zhou J, Yang XR, Qiu SJ, et al. Identification of side population cells in human hepatocellular carcinoma cell lines with stepwise metastatic potentials. J Cancer Res Clin Oncol. 2008;134:1155–63.
102. Haraguchi N, Utsunomiya T, Inoue H, Tanaka F, Mimori K, Barnard GF, et al. Characterization of a side population of cancer cells from human gastrointestinal system. Stem Cells. 2006;24:506–13.
103. Artells R, Moreno I, Diaz T, Martinez F, Gel B, Navarro A, et al. Tumour CD133 mRNA expression and clinical outcome in surgically resected colorectal cancer patients. Eur J Cancer. 2010;46:642–9.
104. Salnikov AV, Gladkich J, Moldenhauer G, Volm M, Mattern J, Herr I. CD133 is indicative for a resistance phenotype but does not represent a prognostic marker for survival of non-small cell lung cancer patients. Int J Cancer. 2010;126:950–8.
105. Yamashita T, Honda M, Nakamoto Y, Baba M, Nio K, Hara Y, et al. Discrete nature of EpCAM+ and CD90+ cancer stem cells in human hepatocellular carcinoma. Hepatology. 2013;57:1484–97.
106. Forner A, Llovet JM, Bruix J. Hepatocellular carcinoma. Lancet. 2012;379:1245–55.
107. Marquardt JU, Galle PR, Teufel A. Molecular diagnosis and therapy of hepatocellular carcinoma (HCC): an emerging field for advanced technologies. J Hepatol. 2012;56:267–75.
108. Villanueva A, Llovet JM. Targeted therapies for hepatocellular carcinoma. Gastroenterology. 2011;140:1410–26.
109. Worns MA, Galle PR. Novel inhibitors in development for hepatocellular carcinoma. Expert Opin Investig Drugs. 2010;19:615–29.
110. Bruix J, Qin S, Merle P, Granito A, Huang YH, Bodoky G, et al. Regorafenib for patients with hepatocellular carcinoma who progressed on sorafenib treatment (RESORCE): a randomised, double-blind, placebo-controlled, phase 3 trial. Lancet. 2017;389:56–66.
111. Wilhelm S, Carter C, Lynch M, Lowinger T, Dumas J, Smith RA, et al. Discovery and development of sorafenib: a multikinase inhibitor for treating cancer. Nat Rev Drug Discov. 2006;5:835–44.
112. Wilhelm SM, Carter C, Tang L, Wilkie D, McNabola A, Rong H, et al. BAY 43-9006 exhibits broad spectrum oral antitumor activity and targets the RAF/MEK/ERK pathway and receptor tyrosine kinases involved in tumor progression and angiogenesis. Cancer Res. 2004;64:7099–109.
113. Chan LH, Luk ST, Ma S. Turning hepatic cancer stem cells inside out--a deeper understanding through multiple perspectives. Mol Cells. 2015;38:202–9.
114. Yang Z, Zhang L, Ma A, Liu L, Li J, Gu J, et al. Transient mTOR inhibition facilitates continuous growth of liver tumors by modulating the maintenance of CD133+ cell populations. PLoS One. 2011;6:e28405.
115. Oishi N, Yamashita T, Kaneko S. Molecular biology of liver cancer stem cells. Liver Cancer. 2014;3:71–84.
116. Clevers H. Wnt/beta-catenin signaling in development and disease. Cell. 2006;127:469–80.
117. Gedaly R, Galuppo R, Daily MF, Shah M, Maynard E, Chen C, et al. Targeting the Wnt/beta-catenin signaling pathway in liver cancer stem cells and hepatocellular carcinoma cell lines with FH535. PLoS One. 2014;9:e99272.
118. Mohammed MK, Shao C, Wang J, Wei Q, Wang X, Collier Z, et al. Wnt/beta-catenin signaling plays an ever-expanding role in stem cell self-renewal, tumorigenesis and cancer chemoresistance. Genes Dis. 2016;3:11–40.
119. Cavard C, Colnot S, Audard V, Benhamouche S, Finzi L, Torre C, et al. Wnt/beta-catenin pathway in hepatocellular carcinoma pathogenesis and liver physiology. Future Oncol. 2008;4:647–60.
120. Ji J, Yamashita T, Budhu A, Forgues M, Jia HL, Li C, et al. Identification of microRNA-181 by genome-wide screening as a critical player in EpCAM-positive hepatic cancer stem cells. Hepatology. 2009;50:472–80.

121. Ji J, Yamashita T, Wang XW. Wnt/beta-catenin signaling activates microRNA-181 expression in hepatocellular carcinoma. Cell Biosci. 2011;1:4.
122. Mokkapati S, Niopek K, Huang L, Cunniff KJ, Ruteshouser EC, deCaestecker M, et al. beta-catenin activation in a novel liver progenitor cell type is sufficient to cause hepatocellular carcinoma and hepatoblastoma. Cancer Res. 2014;74:4515–25.
123. Pez F, Lopez A, Kim M, Wands JR, Caron de Fromentel C, Merle P. Wnt signaling and hepatocarcinogenesis: molecular targets for the development of innovative anticancer drugs. J Hepatol. 2013;59:1107–17.
124. Massague J. TGFbeta signalling in context. Nat Rev Mol Cell Biol. 2012;13:616–30.
125. Inman GJ. Switching TGFbeta from a tumor suppressor to a tumor promoter. Curr Opin Genet Dev. 2011;21:93–9.
126. Bogaerts E, Heindryckx F, Vandewynckel YP, Van Grunsven LA, Van Vlierberghe H. The roles of transforming growth factor-beta, Wnt, Notch and hypoxia on liver progenitor cells in primary liver tumours (Review). Int J Oncol. 2014;44:1015–22.
127. Wu K, Ding J, Chen C, Sun W, Ning BF, Wen W, et al. Hepatic transforming growth factor beta gives rise to tumor-initiating cells and promotes liver cancer development. Hepatology. 2012;56:2255–67.
128. Fernando J, Malfettone A, Cepeda EB, Vilarrasa-Blasi R, Bertran E, Raimondi G, et al. A mesenchymal-like phenotype and expression of CD44 predict lack of apoptotic response to sorafenib in liver tumor cells. Int J Cancer. 2015;136:E161–72.
129. Budhu A, Wang XW. Transforming the microenvironment: a trick of the metastatic cancer cell. Cancer Cell. 2012;22:279–80.
130. Villanueva A, Chiang DY, Newell P, Peix J, Thung S, Alsinet C, et al. Pivotal role of mTOR signaling in hepatocellular carcinoma. Gastroenterology. 2008;1972-1983(1983):135.
131. Lau CK, Yang ZF, Ho DW, Ng MN, Yeoh GC, Poon RT, et al. An Akt/hypoxia-inducible factor-1alpha/platelet-derived growth factor-BB autocrine loop mediates hypoxia-induced chemoresistance in liver cancer cells and tumorigenic hepatic progenitor cells. Clin Cancer Res. 2009;15:3462–71.
132. Villanueva A, Alsinet C, Yanger K, Hoshida Y, Zong Y, Toffanin S, et al. Notch signaling is activated in human hepatocellular carcinoma and induces tumor formation in mice. Gastroenterology. 2012;143:1660–9.e7.
133. Santagata S, Demichelis F, Riva A, Varambally S, Hofer MD, Kutok JL, et al. JAGGED1 expression is associated with prostate cancer metastasis and recurrence. Cancer Res. 2004;64:6854–7.
134. Westhoff B, Colaluca IN, D'Ario G, Donzelli M, Tosoni D, Volorio S, et al. Alterations of the Notch pathway in lung cancer. Proc Natl Acad Sci U S A. 2009;106:22293–8.
135. Viatour P, Ehmer U, Saddic LA, Dorrell C, Andersen JB, Lin C, et al. Notch signaling inhibits hepatocellular carcinoma following inactivation of the RB pathway. J Exp Med. 2011;208:1963–76.
136. Cheng T. Cell cycle inhibitors in normal and tumor stem cells. Oncogene. 2004;23:7256–66.
137. Hooper JE, Scott MP. Communicating with Hedgehogs. Nat Rev Mol Cell Biol. 2005;6:306–17.
138. Varjosalo M, Taipale J. Hedgehog: functions and mechanisms. Genes Dev. 2008;22:2454–72.
139. Omenetti A, Choi S, Michelotti G, Diehl AM. Hedgehog signaling in the liver. J Hepatol. 2011;54:366–73.
140. Varjosalo M, Li SP, Taipale J. Divergence of hedgehog signal transduction mechanism between Drosophila and mammals. Dev Cell. 2006;10:177–86.
141. Omenetti A, Diehl AM. The adventures of sonic hedgehog in development and repair. II. Sonic hedgehog and liver development, inflammation, and cancer. Am J Physiol Gastrointest Liver Physiol. 2008;294:G595–8.
142. Sicklick JK, Li YX, Jayaraman A, Kannangai R, Qi Y, Vivekanandan P, et al. Dysregulation of the Hedgehog pathway in human hepatocarcinogenesis. Carcinogenesis. 2006;27:748–57.
143. Chung SI, Moon H, Ju HL, Cho KJ, Kim do Y, Han KH, et al. Hepatic expression of Sonic Hedgehog induces liver fibrosis and promotes hepatocarcinogenesis in a transgenic mouse model. J Hepatol. 2016;64:618–27.

144. Giakoustidis A, Giakoustidis D, Mudan S, Sklavos A, Williams R. Molecular signalling in hepatocellular carcinoma: Role of and crosstalk among WNT/ss-catenin, Sonic Hedgehog, Notch and Dickkopf-1. Can J Gastroenterol Hepatol. 2015;29:209–17.
145. Huang S, He J, Zhang X, Bian Y, Yang L, Xie G, et al. Activation of the hedgehog pathway in human hepatocellular carcinomas. Carcinogenesis. 2006;27:1334–40.
146. Wang XQ, Ongkeko WM, Chen L, Yang ZF, Lu P, Chen KK, et al. Octamer 4 (Oct4) mediates chemotherapeutic drug resistance in liver cancer cells through a potential Oct4-AKT-ATP-binding cassette G2 pathway. Hepatology. 2010;52:528–39.
147. Sukowati CH, Rosso N, Pascut D, Anfuso B, Torre G, Francalanci P, et al. Gene and functional up-regulation of the BCRP/ABCG2 transporter in hepatocellular carcinoma. BMC Gastroenterol. 2012;12:160.
148. Hatziapostolou M, Polytarchou C, Aggelidou E, Drakaki A, Poultsides GA, Jaeger SA, et al. An HNF4alpha-miRNA inflammatory feedback circuit regulates hepatocellular oncogenesis. Cell. 2011;147:1233–47.
149. Yin C, Lin Y, Zhang X, Chen YX, Zeng X, Yue HY, et al. Differentiation therapy of hepatocellular carcinoma in mice with recombinant adenovirus carrying hepatocyte nuclear factor-4alpha gene. Hepatology. 2008;48:1528–39.
150. Hanahan D, Weinberg RA. Hallmarks of cancer: the next generation. Cell. 2011;144:646–74.
151. Feinberg AP, Tycko B. The history of cancer epigenetics. Nat Rev Cancer. 2004;4:143–53.
152. Lee S, Lee HJ, Kim JH, Lee HS, Jang JJ, Kang GH. Aberrant CpG island hypermethylation along multistep hepatocarcinogenesis. Am J Pathol. 2003;163:1371–8.
153. Wang XQ, Ng RK, Ming X, Zhang W, Chen L, Chu AC, et al. Epigenetic regulation of pluripotent genes mediates stem cell features in human hepatocellular carcinoma and cancer cell lines. PLoS One. 2013;8:e72435.
154. Bitzer M, Horger M, Giannini EG, Ganten TM, Worns MA, Siveke JT, et al. Resminostat in combination with sorafenib as second-line therapy of advanced hepatocellular carcinoma – The SHELTER Study. J Hepatol. 2016;65:280–8.
155. Ventura A, Jacks T. MicroRNAs and cancer: short RNAs go a long way. Cell. 2009;136:586–91.
156. Yang X, Ye J, Yan H, Tang Z, Shen J, Zhang J, et al. MiR-491 attenuates cancer stem cells-like properties of hepatocellular carcinoma by inhibition of GIT-1/NF-kappaB-mediated EMT. Tumour Biol. 2016;37:201–9.
157. Rinn JL, Chang HY. Genome regulation by long noncoding RNAs. Annu Rev Biochem. 2012;81:145–66.
158. Wang X, Sun W, Shen W, Xia M, Chen C, Xiang D, et al. Long non-coding RNA DILC regulates liver cancer stem cells via IL-6/STAT3 axis. J Hepatol. 2016;64:1283–94.
159. Tripathi V, Ellis JD, Shen Z, Song DY, Pan Q, Watt AT, et al. The nuclear-retained noncoding RNA MALAT1 regulates alternative splicing by modulating SR splicing factor phosphorylation. Mol Cell. 2010;39:925–38.
160. Yang F, Yi F, Han X, Du Q, Liang Z. MALAT-1 interacts with hnRNP C in cell cycle regulation. FEBS Lett. 2013;587:3175–81.
161. Guerrieri F. Long non-coding RNAs era in liver cancer. World J Hepatol. 2015;7:1971–3.
162. Worns MA, Galle PR. HCC therapies-lessons learned. Nat Rev Gastroenterol Hepatol. 2014;11:447–52.
163. Tovar V, Cornella H, Moeini A, Vidal S, Hoshida Y, Sia D, et al. Tumour initiating cells and IGF/FGF signalling contribute to sorafenib resistance in hepatocellular carcinoma. Gut. 2017;66:530–40.
164. Hu T, Liu S, Breiter DR, Wang F, Tang Y, Sun S. Octamer 4 small interfering RNA results in cancer stem cell-like cell apoptosis. Cancer Res. 2008;68:6533–40.

Clinical and Preclinical Perspectives on Mechanisms of Sorafenib Resistance in Hepatocellular Carcinoma

Chiun Hsu and Ann-Lii Cheng

Abstract The antitumor mechanisms of sorafenib in hepatocellular carcinoma (HCC) may involve complex interactions of signaling pathways in cancer cells and the tumor microenvironment, thus rendering the exploration of strategies to reverse sorafenib resistance an extremely challenging task. This chapter reviews the results of clinical trials of systemic therapy for patients with sorafenib-resistant HCC and preclinical studies exploring mechanisms and biomarkers of sorafenib resistance in HCC. The insights and limitations of these studies are discussed.

Keywords Clinical trials • Drug resistance • Hepatocellular carcinoma • Immunotherapy • Molecular targeted therapy • Preclinical models

Abbreviations

AFP	α-fetoprotein
FGFR	Fibroblast growth factor receptor
HCC	Hepatocellular carcinoma
mTOR	Mammalian target of rapamycin
VEGFR-2	Vascular endothelial growth factor receptor 2

C. Hsu • A.-L. Cheng (✉)
Graduate Institute of Oncology, National Taiwan University College of Medicine, Taipei, Taiwan

Department of Oncology, National Taiwan University Hospital, No. 7, Chung-Shan South Road, Taipei 100, Taiwan

National Taiwan University Cancer Center, Taipei, Taiwan
e-mail: alcheng@ntu.edu.tw

A. Villanueva (ed.), *Resistance to Molecular Therapies for Hepatocellular Carcinoma*, Resistance to Targeted Anti-Cancer Therapeutics,
DOI 10.1007/978-3-319-56197-4_5

Introduction

The multikinase inhibitor sorafenib remains the standard systemic therapy for patients with advanced hepatocellular carcinoma (HCC) because of the survival benefit demonstrated by randomized, placebo-controlled trials [1]. Post-market surveys have confirmed the findings of clinical trials, including a median time-to-tumor progression of 3–5 months, an objective tumor response of 2–3%, and an acceptable safety profile at the recommended dosage of 400 mg twice daily [2, 3]. The aforementioned data clearly indicate the challenge of overcoming sorafenib resistance in patients with HCC.

Sorafenib targets multiple receptors and intracellular kinases, including Raf-1, B-Raf, vascular endothelial growth factor receptor 2 (VEGFR-2), platelet-derived growth factor receptor, and c-Kit, and exhibits both antitumor and antiangiogenic effects [4]. However, many studies have reported that the potential targets of sorafenib involve complex interactions of signaling pathways in cancer cells and the tumor microenvironment. Although such studies have provided insights into the mechanisms of sorafenib resistance, the complex targets of sorafenib in HCC have rendered the exploration of strategies to reverse sorafenib resistance a highly challenging task. Mechanistic exploration for sorafenib resistance in HCC is difficult primarily because of the clinical and molecular heterogeneities of the patient population as well as the paucity of the tumor specimens available for analysis with corresponding efficacy data after sorafenib treatment. Some of these aspects are discussed in other sections of this book. In this chapter, we review the results of clinical and preclinical studies aimed at overcoming sorafenib resistance in HCC. We also discuss the insights and limitations of such studies.

Lessons from Second-Line Clinical Trials in HCC

After the success of trials demonstrating the efficacy of sorafenib as first-line therapy for advanced HCC, many clinical trials have been conducted in the second-line setting to explore the efficacy of targeted agents with various mechanisms of action. Such trials have usually enrolled patients who developed progressive disease after sorafenib treatment. Therefore, the results reflect the clinical features of advanced HCC that are resistant to sorafenib treatment. Table 1 presents a summary of representative studies [5–10].

The first class of the trials have explored novel antiangiogenic therapy. Sorafenib exerts antiangiogenic effects by inhibiting the VEGF signaling pathway, and this is one of the major antitumor mechanisms of sorafenib for HCC. Moreover, agents with more potent antiangiogenic effects were hypothesized to overcome sorafenib resistance in HCC. Axitinib is a selective inhibitor of VEGFR-1–3 in the nanomolar range. Ramucirumab is a recombinant monoclonal antibody that specifically binds to VEGFR-2 with a high affinity. Axitinib and ramucirumab exhibit antitumor

Table 1 Clinical trials of second-line systemic therapy for advanced HCC

Authors (ref)	Treatment (patient no.)	Eligibility	OS (months)	HR (95% C.I.)/ p value	PFS (months)	HR (95% C.I.)/ p value	Remarks
Bruix [14]	Regorafenib (379)	Progression after sorafenib	10.6	0.63 (0.50–0.79)/ <0.0001	3.1	0.46 (0.37–0.56)/ <0.0001	
	Placebo (194)		7.8		1.5		
Llovet [5]	Brivanib (263)	Progression after/intolerance to sorafenib treatment	9.4	0.89 (0.69–1.15)/ 0.33	4.2	0.56 (0.42–0.76)/ <0.001	
	Placebo (132)		8.2		2.7		
Zhu [6]	Ramucirumab (283)	Progression after/intolerance to sorafenib treatment	9.2	0.87 (0.72–1.05)/ 0.14	2.8	0.63 (0.52–0.75)/ 0.001	AFP ≧ 400 ng/ mLmay predict efficacy
	Placebo (282)		7.6		2.1		
Kang [7]	Axitinib (134)	1 prior systemic anti-angiogenic therapy	12.7	0.91 (0.65–1.27)/ 0.29	3.6	0.62 (0.44–0.81)/ 0.004	Asian subjects tended to benefit more from axitinib treatment
	Placebo (68)		9.7		1.9		
Zhu [8]	Everolimus (362)	Progression after/intolerance to sorafenib treatment	7.6	1.05 (0.86–1.27) 0.68	3.0	0.93 (0.75–1.15) NR	HBV(+) subjects tended to benefit from everolimus treatment
	Placebo (184)		7.3		2.6		
Santoro [9]	Tivantinib (71)	1 prior systemic therapy (96% received sorafenib)	6.6	0.90 (0.57–1.40)/ 0.63	1.5	0.67 (0.44–1.04)/ 0.06	Potential benefit for MET-high tumors
	Placebo (36)		6.2		1.4		
Abou-Alfa [10]	Codrituzumab (125)	≥1 prior systemic therapy (79% received sorafenib)	8.7	0.96 (0.65–1.41)/ 0.82	2.6	0.97 (0.67–1.39)/ 0.87	GPC3 expression did not correlate with efficacy
	Placebo (60)		10.0		1.5		

efficacy in patients who developed progressive metastatic renal cell carcinoma after sorafenib treatment [11, 12]. Brivanib can inhibit both VEGFR and fibroblast growth factor receptor (FGFR) signaling, and upregulation of FGFR signaling is a crucial resistance mechanism for anti-VEGFR treatment [13].

Although none of the placebo-controlled trials of the three aforementioned agents demonstrated an overall survival benefit for the experimental therapy, several findings are notable. First, all trials have demonstrated significant improvement of progression-free survival after the experimental therapy, suggesting that agents with more potent antiangiogenic effects are likely to overcome sorafenib resistance in patients with HCC. This hypothesis is further supported by the positive results obtained for regorafenib as second-line therapy for advanced HCC. Based on its kinase inhibition profile, regorafenib is presumed to have more potent antiangiogenic effects than sorafenib does [14, 15]. Second, predictive biomarkers may enable the selection of patients who are most likely to benefit from these new agents. Ramucirumab treatment was associated with a significant overall survival benefit in a subgroup of patients with baseline α-fetoprotein (AFP) levels higher than 400 ng/mL (hazard ratio [HR] 0.67, 95% confidence interval [CI] 0.51–0.90, $p = 0.006$). A similar trend of overall survival benefit was reported for patients with AFP levels higher than 400 ng/mL in the axitinib trial (HR 0.67, 95% CI 0.42–1.07). It was postulated that elevated AFP levels were associated with the upregulation of angiogenesis-related signaling pathways; thus, the high-AFP subgroup may benefit more from more potent antiangiogenic therapy [16]. Another potential approach for selecting patients likely to benefit from more potent antiangiogenic therapy is the use of functional imaging to monitor the vascular response of the tumors after anti-angiogenic therapy [17, 18].

The second class of the trials have explored agents targeting molecules/signaling pathways considered to be involved in hepatocarcinogenesis, cancer progression, or cell survival regulation. Randomized trials of everolimus (mammalian target of rapamycin [mTOR] inhibitor), tivantinib (c-met inhibitor), and codrituzumab (anti-glypican-3 antibody) all failed to demonstrate significant improvements in overall survival compared with placebo. Although subgroup analysis showed a potential benefit in selected patient subgroups, an adequate interpretation of the results is more complicated. In the everolimus trial, patients with hepatitis B virus infection may have improved overall survival after everolimus treatment (HR 0.64, 95% CI 0.45–0.93). The biological rationale underlying this phenomenon is unknown. In the tivantinib phase 2b trial, patients with high c-MET, defined by immunochemical staining of ≥2+ in ≥50% of tumor cells, had longer time-to-tumor progression after tivantinib treatment, compared with patients with low c-MET (2.7 vs. 1.4 months, HR 0.43, 95% CI 0.19–0.97, $p = 0.03$). However, tivantinib may exert its antitumor effects independent of its inhibitory activity on c-MET, thus rendering the correlation between the c-MET status of the cancer cells and clinical efficacy more questionable [19]. In addition, although the predictive value of c-met expression has been suggested by trials testing c-MET inhibitors in other cancer types, the results are inconsistent. Validation from prospective studies targeting a selected patient population is still required [20, 21]. In the codrituzumab trial, longer progression-free survival was observed in patients with higher drug exposure, defined by the trough drug concentration after two cycles of codrituzumab treatment. A hypothesis indicated that a high drug concentration is required to elicit the antitumor response of the host's natural killer cells through antibody-dependent cytotoxicity, but direct pharmacodynamic evidence is lacking.

The aforementioned failed trials reflect the common challenges in developing new drug therapy to overcome sorafenib resistance. The first is the clinical variability of the patient population. Patients in the placebo group of these second-line trials exhibited variable survival times, between 6 and 10 months, which were much longer than those expected when the trials were initially designed. Future studies in the second-line setting should avoid the confounding effects of patients' clinical characteristics and the potential imbalance of post-progression therapy between treatment groups [22, 23]. The second is the lack of a dominant antitumor mechanism of sorafenib and reliable biomarkers predicting treatment efficacy. Therefore, the selection of agents, either as single-agent therapy in the second-line setting or as sorafenib-based combination therapy in the first-line setting, is based on extremely limited preclinical and clinical evidences. Trials combining sorafenib with everolimus (mTOR inhibitor), erlotinib (epidermal growth factor receptor inhibitor), or tigatuzumab (anti-death receptor-5 antibody) all suffered from the same problem [24–26].

Preclinical and Translational Data on Mechanisms of Sorafenib Resistance

Preclinical and translational studies exploring the issue of sorafenib resistance can be categorized into two groups. The first type involves studies that have measured biomarkers by using blood or tissue samples obtained from patients who received sorafenib treatment and correlated the marker status with treatment efficacy. The second type involves studies that have used cell lines or animal models to mimic the development of sorafenib resistance to identify molecular mechanisms of resistance. Studies using these two approaches have been comprehensively reviewed recently [27, 28].

Theoretically, biomarker studies are most valuable when they are incorporated into new drug clinical trials. However, because clinical diagnosis is widely accepted for HCC, tissue samples are available for less than half of the patients enrolled into clinical trials of targeted therapy. An alternative approach is to characterize the molecular features of patients with an excellent response to targeted therapy. Examples of this approach include the identification of FGF3/FGF4 amplification as a marker of the efficacy of sorafenib and loss of tuberous sclerosis complex 2 as a marker of the efficacy of everolimus [29, 30]. Genetic markers are more robust, whereas the measurement of the expression and phosphorylation status of protein markers is subject to multiple technical challenges [31]. Furthermore, a single tumor biopsy specimen may not represent the whole genetic landscape of a patient because synchronous multifocal tumors of different clonality or intra-tumor heterogeneity are common in HCC [32]. Whether detecting circulating tumor cells or tumor-free DNA can resolve this issue is unclear [33].

Biomarkers derived from blood samples are easy to obtain and can be followed up serially after drug treatment. Most studies have applied an arbitrary cutoff value and compared the treatment outcome among subgroups (e.g., patients with a biomarker above or below the median values or patients in different quartiles) [34–36]. Therefore, the external validity of the results is limited. In many studies, data were derived from a single treatment group, and the prognostic versus predictive value of a specific biomarker must be carefully evaluated. Despite these limitations, studies of patients with HCC who received sorafenib as systemic therapy have suggested the following predictors of sorafenib resistance: high baseline levels of angiopoietin-2, hepatocyte growth factor, or transforming growth factor-β1, and low levels of c-kit or insulin-like growth factor-1. These factors, which encompass the regulation of a wide spectrum of malignant phenotypes of aberrant cell growth, angiogenesis, inflammation, and metastases, may reflect the multifaceted action of sorafenib on cancer cells and the tumor microenvironment.

Studies using preclinical cell lines and animal models to investigate the mechanisms of sorafenib resistance in HCC have explored every aspect of "the hallmarks of cancer," again illustrating the multifaceted action of sorafenib [37]. Development of sorafenib resistance in HCC has been linked to aberrant proliferative signaling [38, 39], evasion from growth suppressors or cell death signals [40–42], replicative immortality [43], abnormal angiogenesis [44], invasion and metastasis potential [45, 46], reprogramming of energy metabolism [47], and evading immune destruction (Table 2) [48, 49]. The findings of these studies should be interpreted with caution, particularly when they are used as rationale for designing clinical trials of combination therapy. First, the sorafenib resistance phenotypes defined in these studies are mostly "relative"; that is, the IC50 of sorafenib of the resistant cell lines is only two- to five-fold that of "sensitive" parental cell lines. The distinction of the biomarkers between resistant and sensitive cells is quantitative (increased or decreased levels of expression) rather than qualitative (e.g., occurrence of new mutations). Second, the resistance biomarkers identified by cell line and animal studies generally have not been externally validated, and the effect size of drug treatment has often been overestimated [50]. Third, the animal models of liver cancer generated by inducing specific oncogenes may not recapitulate the real hepatocarcinogenesis process. The relevance of animal models in the development of new drug therapy will be even more challenging in the new era of cancer immunotherapy.

Future Perspectives

Advances in systemic therapy for advanced HCC after the success of sorafenib have been slow. Moreover, current understanding of the mechanisms of sorafenib resistance in HCC remains fragmented. Currently, there is a paradigm shift of systemic

Table 2 Preclinical models exploring mechanisms of sorafenib resistance in HCC

Phenotypes associated with sorafenib resistance	Author (ref)	Major findings	Model used
Aberrant proliferative signaling	Rudalska et al. [38]	Mapk14 (p38a) activation, which led to activation of Mek-Erk and Atf2 signaling, conferred resistance to sorafenib	Multifocal HCCs induced by transposon-based delivery of oncogenic NrasG12V (using the pCaN vector) into the livers of p19Arf-deficient mice
	Hsu et al. [39]	Overexpression of cyclin E1 and downstream Mcl-1 contributed to sorafenib resistance	In vitro induction of sorafenib resistance by exposure of HCC cells to increasing concentration (up to 10 μM) of sorafenib in culture. Xenograft mouse models
Evasion from growth suppressors or cell death signals	Ou et al. [40]	ERK activation and phosphorylation/degradation of the pro-apoptotic BIM was associated with sorafenib resistance	In vitro induction of sorafenib resistance by exposure of HCC cells to increasing concentration (up to 10 μM) of sorafenib in culture. Xenograft mouse models
	Chen et al. [41]	Activation of PI3K/Akt signaling pathway mediates acquired resistance to sorafenib in HCC	
	Ou et al. [42]	GADD45γ (Growth arrest DNA damage-inducible gene γ) suppression is a poor prognostic factor in patients with HCC and may help predict sorafenib efficacy in HCC	
Replicative immortality	Hagiwara et al. [43]	JNK activity in HCC cells correlated with CD133 expression level and inferior response to sorafenib	Human HCC cell lines (Huh7 and HepG2) Xenograft mouse models
Abnormal angiogenesis	Horwitz et al. [44]	*VEGFA* amplification is a potential biomarker for HCC response to sorafenib and other inhibitors of VEGF signaling	*Mdr2* -deficient mice that can develop chronic liver inflammation and eventually liver tumors

(continued)

Table 2 (continued)

Phenotypes associated with sorafenib resistance	Author (ref)	Major findings	Model used
Invasion and metastasis potential	Chen et al. [45]	Poorly-differentiated hepatoma cells, which were characterized by epithelial-mesenchymal transition and enhanced hedgehog signaling activity, were more invasive and resistant to sorafenib and cytotoxic agents	6 human HCC cell lines Xenograft mouse models
	Fernando et al. [46]	Mesenchymal phenotype, expression of CD44, and activation of the TGF-b pathway, may predict lack of response to sorafenib	6 human HCC cell lines Xenograft mouse models
Reprogramming of energy metabolism	Shen et al. [47]	Extent of aerobic glycolysis correlated with sorafenib resistance, which can be reversed by treatment with the pyruvate dehydrogenase kinase inhibitor, dichloroacetate	In vitro induction of sorafenib resistance by exposure of HCC cells to increasing concentration (up to 10 μM) of sorafenib in culture. Xenograft mouse models
Evading immune destruction	Chen et al. [48]	Sorafenib increased stromal-derived factor 1 alpha (SDF-1α) expression, and SDF-1α/C-X-C receptor type 4 (CXCR4) activation promotes hepatic stellate cell (HSC) differentiation, tumor fibrosis, and drug resistance	Orthotopic implantation of HCA-1 mouse liver cancer cell lines into C3H or Mst1−/−Mst2F/− mice treated with CCl4 (to induce liver fibrosis)
	Chang et al. [49]	Sorafenib increased the intratumor infiltration of CD11b + Gr1 + Ly6G + Ly6Clo myeloid-derived suppressor cells, which may impaired the therapeutic efficacy of sorafenib through promoting immune-suppression and angiogenesis	Orthotopic implantation of BNL 1MEA.7R.1 mouse liver cancer cell lines into BALB/c mice

anticancer therapy from molecular targeted therapy to immunotherapy. Immune checkpoint inhibitor therapy, which has revolutionized systemic therapy for multiple cancer types, is also promising for advanced HCC [51] The insight gained from the mechanistic and biomarker studies of sorafenib in HCC will serve as a solid basis for future exploration of immunotherapy and combination therapy.

Acknowledgement This article was supported by grants from the Ministry of Science and Technology, Taiwan (NSC 102-2314-B-002 -142 -MY3, NSC 101-2321-B-002 -014, MOST 103-2314-B-002 -112 -MY3, MOST 105-2314-B-002-199).

Conflict of Interest Statement Prof. Ann-Lii Cheng is a consultant for Novartis, Eisai, Merck Serono, Merck Sharp & Dohme, and Bayer.

References

1. Forner A, Llovet JM, Bruix J. Hepatocellular carcinoma. Lancet. 2012;379:1245–55.
2. Lencioni R, Kudo M, Ye SL, et al. GIDEON (Global Investigation of therapeutic DEcisions in hepatocellular carcinoma and Of its treatment with sorafeNib): second interim analysis. Int J Clin Pract. 2014;68:609–17.
3. Iavarone M, Cabibbo G, Piscaglia F, et al. Field-practice study of sorafenib therapy for hepatocellular carcinoma: a prospective multicenter study in Italy. Hepatology. 2011;54:2055–63.
4. Wilhelm SM, Adnane L, Newell P, et al. Preclinical overview of sorafenib, a multikinase inhibitor that targets both Raf and VEGF and PDGF receptor tyrosine kinase signaling. Mol Cancer Ther. 2008;7:3129–40.
5. Llovet JM, Decaens T, Raoul JL, et al. Brivanib in patients with advanced hepatocellular carcinoma who were intolerant to sorafenib or for whom sorafenib failed: results from the randomized phase III BRISK-PS study. J Clin Oncol. 2013;31:3509–16.
6. Zhu AX, Park JO, Ryoo BY, et al. Ramucirumab versus placebo as second-line treatment in patients with advanced hepatocellular carcinoma following first-line therapy with sorafenib (REACH): a randomised, double-blind, multicentre, phase 3 trial. Lancet Oncol. 2015;16:859–70.
7. Kang YK, Yau T, Park JW, et al. Randomized phase II study of axitinib versus placebo plus best supportive care in second-line treatment of advanced hepatocellular carcinoma. Ann Oncol. 2015;26:2457–63.
8. Zhu AX, Kudo M, Assenat E, et al. Effect of everolimus on survival in advanced hepatocellular carcinoma after failure of sorafenib: the EVOLVE-1 randomized clinical trial. JAMA. 2014;312:57 67.
9. Santoro A, Rimassa L, Borbath I, et al. Tivantinib for second-line treatment of advanced hepatocellular carcinoma: a randomised, placebo-controlled phase 2 study. Lancet Oncol. 2013;14:55–63.
10. Abou-Alfa GK, Puig O, Daniele B, et al. Randomized Phase II placebo controlled study of codrituzumab in previously treated patients with advanced hepatocellular carcinoma. J Hepatol. 2016;65(2):289–95. doi:10.1016/j.jhep.2016.04.004.
11. Motzer RJ, Escudier B, Tomczak P, et al. Axitinib versus sorafenib as second-line treatment for advanced renal cell carcinoma: overall survival analysis and updated results from a randomised phase 3 trial. Lancet Oncol. 2013;14:552–62.
12. Garcia JA, Hudes GR, Choueiri TK, et al. A phase 2, single-arm study of ramucirumab in patients with metastatic renal cell carcinoma with disease progression on or intolerance to tyrosine kinase inhibitor therapy. Cancer. 2014;120:1647–55.

13. Finn RS, Kang YK, Mulcahy M, et al. Phase II, open-label study of brivanib as second-line therapy in patients with advanced hepatocellular carcinoma. Clin Cancer Res. 2012;18:2090–8.
14. Bruix J, Qin S, Merle P, et al. Regorafenib for patients with hepatocellular carcinoma who progressed on sorafenib treatment (RESORCE): a randomised, double-blind, placebo-controlled, phase 3 trial. Lancet. 2016; doi:10.1016/S0140-6736(16)32453-9. (Epub ahead of print)
15. Chan SL, Ma BB. An update on the safety and efficacy of regorafenib in the treatment of solid cancers. Expert Opin Drug Metab Toxicol. 2014;10:1607–14.
16. Hoshida Y, Nijman SM, Kobayashi M, et al. Integrative transcriptome analysis reveals common molecular subclasses of human hepatocellular carcinoma. Cancer Res. 2009;69:7385–92.
17. Lo GM, Al Zahrani H, Jang HJ, et al. Detection of early tumor response to axitinib in advanced hepatocellular carcinoma by dynamic contrast enhanced ultrasound. Ultrasound Med Biol. 2016;42:1303–11.
18. Hsu CY, Shen YC, Yu CW, et al. Dynamic contrast-enhanced magnetic resonance imaging biomarkers predict survival and response in hepatocellular carcinoma patients treated with sorafenib and metronomic tegafur/uracil. J Hepatol. 2011;55:858–65.
19. Basilico C, Pennacchietti S, Vigna E, et al. Tivantinib (ARQ197) displays cytotoxic activity that is independent of its ability to bind MET. Clin Cancer Res. 2013;19:2381–92.
20. Scagliotti GV, Di Maio M. Tivantinib added to erlotinib in nonsmall-cell lung cancer: the primary end point was not MET…. Ann Oncol. 2015;26:2007–9.
21. Eng C, Bessudo A, Hart LL, et al. A randomized, placebo-controlled, phase 1/2 study of tivantinib (ARQ 197) in combination with irinotecan and cetuximab in patients with metastatic colorectal cancer with wild-type KRAS who have received first-line systemic therapy. Int J Cancer. 2016;139:177–86.
22. Kelly RK. Brivanib and FOLFOX in hepatocellular carcinoma: finding the common themes among negative trials. J Clin Oncol. 2013;31:3483–6.
23. Shao YY, Wu CH, Lu LC, et al. Prognosis of patients with advanced hepatocellular carcinoma who failed first-line systemic therapy. J Hepatol. 2014;60:313–8.
24. Koeberle D, Dufour JF, Demeter G, et al. Sorafenib with or without everolimus in patients with advanced hepatocellular carcinoma (HCC): a randomized multicenter, multinational phase II trial (SAKK 77/08 and SASL 29). Ann Oncol. 2016;27:856–61.
25. Zhu AX, Rosmorduc O, Evans TR, et al. SEARCH: a phase III, randomized, double-blind, placebo-controlled trial of sorafenib plus erlotinib in patients with advanced hepatocellular carcinoma. J Clin Oncol. 2015;33:559–66.
26. Cheng AL, Kang YK, He AR, et al. Safety and efficacy of tigatuzumab plus sorafenib as first-line therapy in subjects with advanced hepatocellular carcinoma: a phase 2 randomized study. J Hepatol. 2015;63:896–904.
27. Shao YY, Hsu CH, Cheng AL. Predictive biomarkers of sorafenib efficacy in advanced hepatocellular carcinoma: are we getting there? World J Gastroenterol. 2015;21:10336–47.
28. Nishida N, Kitano M, Sakurai T, et al. Molecular mechanism and prediction of sorafenib chemoresistance in human hepatocellular carcinoma. Dig Dis. 2015;33:771–9.
29. Arao T, Ueshima K, Matsumoto K, et al. FGF3/FGF4 amplification and multiple lung metastases in responders to sorafenib in hepatocellular carcinoma. Hepatology. 2013;57:1407–15.
30. Huynh H, Hao HX, Chan SL, et al. Loss of tuberous sclerosis complex 2 (TSC2) is frequent in hepatocellular carcinoma and predicts response to mTORC1 inhibitor everolimus. Mol Cancer Ther. 2015;14:1224–35.
31. Shao YY, Chen CL, Ho MC, et al. Dissimilar immunohistochemical expression of ERK and AKT between paired biopsy and hepatectomy tissues of hepatocellular carcinoma. Anticancer Res. 2012;32:4865–70.
32. Lu LC, Hsu CH, Hsu C, et al. Tumor heterogeneity in hepatocellular carcinoma: facing the challenges. Liver Cancer. 2016;5:128–38.
33. Chan SL, Wong AM, Lee K, Wong N, Chan AK. Personalized therapy for hepatocellular carcinoma: where are we now? Cancer Treat Rev. 2016;45:77–86.
34. Llovet JM, Peña CE, Lathia CD, et al. Plasma biomarkers as predictors of outcome in patients with advanced hepatocellular carcinoma. Clin Cancer Res. 2012;18:2290–300.

35. Zhu AX, Kang YK, Rosmorduc O, et al. Biomarker analyses of clinical outcomes in patients with advanced hepatocellular carcinoma treated with sorafenib with or without erlotinib in the SEARCH trial. Clin Cancer Res. 2016;22(19):4870–9. Epub 2016 May 24
36. Lin TH, Shao YY, Chan SY, et al. High serum transforming growth factor-β1 levels predict outcome in hepatocellular carcinoma patients treated with sorafenib. Clin Cancer Res. 2015;21:3678–84.
37. Hanahan D, Weinberg RA. Hallmarks of cancer: the next generation. Cell. 2011;144:646–74.
38. Rudalska R, Dauch D, Longerich T, et al. In vivo RNAi screening identifies a mechanism of sorafenib resistance in liver cancer. Nat Med. 2014;20:1138–46.
39. Hsu C, Lin LI, Cheng YC, et al. Cyclin E1 inhibition can overcome sorafenib resistance in hepatocellular carcinoma cells through Mcl-1 suppression. Clin Cancer Res. 2016;22:2555–64.
40. Ou DL, Shen YC, Liang JD, et al. Induction of Bim expression contributes to the anti-tumor synergy between sorafenib and the MEK Inhibitor CI-1040 in hepatocellular carcinoma. Clin Cancer Res. 2009;15:5820–8.
41. Chen KF, Chen HL, Tai WT, et al. Activation of phosphatidylinositol 3-kinase/Akt signaling pathway mediates acquired resistance to sorafenib in hepatocellular carcinoma cells. J Pharmacol Exp Ther. 2011;337:155–61.
42. Ou DL, Shyue SK, Lin LI, et al. Growth arrest DNA damage-inducible gene 45 gamma expression as a prognostic and predictive biomarker in hepatocellular carcinoma. Oncotarget. 2015;6:27953–65.
43. Hagiwara S, Kudo M, Nagai T, et al. Activation of JNK and high expression level of CD133 predict a poor response to sorafenib in hepatocellular carcinoma. Br J Cancer. 2012;106:1997–2003.
44. Horwitz E, Stein I, Andreozzi M, et al. Human and mouse *VEGFA*-amplified hepatocellular carcinomas are highly sensitive to sorafenib treatment. Cancer Discov. 2014;4:730–43.
45. Chen X, Lingala S, Khoobyari S, et al. Epithelial mesenchymal transition and hedgehog signaling activation are associated with chemoresistance and invasion of hepatoma subpopulations. J Hepatol. 2011;55:838–45.
46. Fernando J, Malfettone A, Cepeda EB, et al. A mesenchymal-like phenotype and expression of CD44 predict lack of apoptotic response to sorafenib in liver tumor cells. Int J Cancer. 2015;136:E161–72.
47. Shen YC, Ou DL, Hsu C, et al. Activating oxidative phosphorylation by a pyruvate dehydrogenase kinase inhibitor overcomes sorafenib resistance of hepatocellular carcinoma. Br J Cancer. 2013;108:72–81.
48. Chen Y, Ramjiawan RR, Reiberger T, et al. Differential effects of sorafenib on liver versus tumor fibrosis mediated by stromal-derived factor 1 alpha/C-X-C receptor type 4 axis and myeloid differentiation antigen–positive myeloid cell infiltration in mice. Hepatology. 2014;59:1435–47.
49. Chang CJ, Yang YH, Chiu CJ, et al. Therapeutic effect of sorafenib is attenuated by tumor-infiltrating Ly6G+ myeloid-derived suppressor cells (MDSCs) and is restored by anti-interleukin-6 (IL-6) antibody treatment in an orthotopic mouse liver cancer model. Proc Am Assoc Cancer Res 2015; abstr#461.
50. Mattina J, MacKinnon N, Henderson VC, et al. Design and reporting of targeted anticancer preclinical studies: a meta-analysis of animal studies investigating sorafenib antitumor efficacy. Cancer Res. 2016;76(16):4627–36. doi:10.1158/0008-5472.CAN-15-3455.
51. Sangro B, Melero I, Yau T, et al. Safety and antitumor activity of nivolumab (nivo) in patients (pts) with advanced hepatocellular carcinoma (HCC): interim analysis of dose-expansion cohorts from the phase 1/2 CheckMate-040 study. ASCO 2016; abstr no. 4012.

Radiological Assessment of Response to Palliative Treatments in Hepatocellular Carcinoma

Riccardo Lencioni

Abstract Assessment of hepatocellular carcinoma (HCC) response to palliative treatment entails unique complexities and requires adequate background and skills for proper image interpretation. Modified RECIST (mRECIST) criteria incorporate HCC-specific amendments to standard RECIST and are currently endorsed by both the EASL-EORTC and the ESMO-ESDO guidelines. It has been shown that patients with mRECIST response after loco-regional therapies have longer survival than non-responders. However, the data are still limited for systemic therapies. Also, the pattern of tumor progression may have major implications for patient management and post-progression survival prediction. With the advent of immune checkpoint inhibitors, the basic structure of the RECIST model might require substantial changes. Finally, caution should be exercised in translating response assessment models developed for clinical trials into clinical practice.

Keywords Hepatocellular carcinoma • Modified RECIST • mRECIST • Sorafenib

Abbreviations

AASLD	American Association for the Study of Liver Diseases
CR	Complete response
CT	Computed tomography
EASL	European Association for the Study of the Liver
EORTC	European Organization for Research and Treatment of Cancer
ESDO	European Society of Digestive Oncology
ESMO	European Society of Medical Oncology

R. Lencioni (✉)
Clinical and Translational Research, Sylvester Comprehensive Cancer Center, 1475 NW 12th Avenue, Miami, FL 33149, USA

Department of Interventional Radiology, University of Miami Miller School of Medicine, Miami, FL, USA
e-mail: rlencioni@med.miami.edu

A. Villanueva (ed.), *Resistance to Molecular Therapies for Hepatocellular Carcinoma*, Resistance to Targeted Anti-Cancer Therapeutics,
DOI 10.1007/978-3-319-56197-4_6

HCC	Hepatocellular carcinoma
MRI	Magnetic resonance imaging
PD	Progressive disease
PR	Partial response
RECIST	Response Evaluation Criteria in Solid Tumors
SD	Stable disease
TACE	Transcatheter arterial chemoembolization
TTP	Time to progression
WHO	World Health Organization

Introduction

Tumor response in oncology is typically measured according to Response Evaluation Criteria in Solid Tumors (RECIST). The RECIST guideline defines standard measurement methods for converting radiology image observations into a quantitative and statistically tractable framework for measuring tumor response. The RECIST model—developed in 2000 and revised in 2009—was designed for the evaluation of cytotoxic agents [1, 2]. It offers a simple approach to determining lesion size changes during treatment as an indicator of response. However, it does not address measures of antitumor activity other than tumor shrinkage. In fact, the RECIST document acknowledges that amendments to the general guideline could be needed for the evaluation of other anticancer therapies as well as for the assessment of tumors presenting unique complexities [1, 2].

In the case of hepatocellular carcinoma (HCC), statistically significant and clinically meaningful improvements in survival were observed in patients receiving liver-directed or molecular targeted therapies in the absence of substantial tumor reduction as assessed by using standard RECIST [3–5]. Given the poor correlation between response evaluation by conventional metrics and overall survival outcomes, a group of experts convened by the American Association for the Study of Liver Diseases (AASLD) proposed specific amendments to standard RECIST [6]. The resulting criteria were named modified RECIST (mRECIST) for HCC [7]. The mRECIST model is based on the recommendations for image interpretation developed as part of the Radiology Charter of the SHARP trial [3] to prevent incorrect diagnoses of progression resulting from the strict application of standard RECIST and incorporates the concept of viable tumor already proposed in the 2000 EASL guidelines on the management of HCC.

The mRECIST criteria are currently endorsed by several scientific societies and organizations, including the European Association for the Study of the Liver (EASL), the European Organization for Research and Treatment of Cancer (EORTC), the European Society of Medical Oncology (ESMO), and the European Society of Digestive Oncology (ESDO) [8, 9]. However, further validation has been recommended to understand the outcome prediction capability in patients receiving different forms of loco-regional or systemic treatment. This chapter reviews basic principles of the mRECIST methodology and discuss available data and open questions in the evaluation of tumor response and progression.

mRECIST Assessment at Baseline

Tumor lesions are categorized at baseline as either measurable or non-measurable. Measurable lesions include lesions that can be accurately measured in at least one dimension as ≥1 cm with computed tomography (CT) or magnetic resonance imaging (MRI). Non-measurable lesions include small lesions (longest diameter <1 cm with CT or MRI) and truly non-measurable lesions such as malignant effusions. Measurable lesions up to a maximum of two lesions per organ and five lesions in total (or five lesions per organ and ten lesions in total), suitable for accurate and repeat measurement, may be selected as target lesions and measured at baseline. All other lesions (or sites of disease) should be identified as non-target lesions. In the selection of the target lesions, priority should be given to intrahepatic HCC nodules that show intratumoral arterial enhancement at contrast-enhanced CT or MRI.

The baseline sum diameter of the target lesions, to which any subsequent measurements will be compared for the determination of response, is obtained by the sum of the longest diameters of each target lesion. Of importance, the mRECIST guideline has introduced the concept of viable tumor for the measurement of intrahepatic HCC nodules with typical vascular profile. According to mRECIST, it is the longest diameter of the viable portion of the tumor, not the longest overall tumor diameter, that has to be measured. Therefore, areas of internal necrosis (either spontaneous necrosis or necrosis induced by prior interventions) should not be included in the measurement.

All tumor lesions (or sites of disease) that have not been selected as target lesions should be identified as non-target lesions and should also be recorded at baseline. Measurements of non-target lesions are not required, but the presence or absence of each should be noted throughout follow-up. Infiltrative-type HCC should be considered as a non-target lesion when the mass shows ill-defined borders and therefore does not appear to be suitable for accurate and repeat measurements. Malignant portal vein thrombosis should also be considered as a non-target lesion due to the difficulty in performing consistent repeat measurements of the malignant thrombus. Of note, ascites and pleural effusion should not be considered as tumor lesions unless associated with clear-cut neoplastic peritoneal or pleural nodules or when cytology confirmation of their malignant nature is available.

mRECIST Evaluation of Tumor Response

The overall patient response at a given post-baseline timepoint is the result of the combined assessment of target lesions and non-target lesions response. In addition, the overall patient response is dependent on the presence or absence of new tumor lesions (Table 1).

Table 1 mRECIST assessment of tumor response: overall responses for all possible combinations of tumor response in target and non-target lesions with or without the appearance of new lesions (adapted from [2])

Target lesions	Non-target lesions	New lesions	Overall response
CR	CR	No	CR
CR	IR/SD	No	PR
PR	Non-PD	No	PR
SD	Non-PD	No	SD
PD	Any	Yes or no	PD
Any	PD	Yes or no	PD
Any	Any	Yes	PD

CR complete response, *PR* partial response, *SD* stable disease, *IR* incomplete response, *PD* progressive disease

According to mRECIST, the sum diameter of the target lesions at each post-baseline timepoint is obtained by the sum of the longest diameter of the viable portion of intrahepatic target lesions with typical vascular profile at baseline, plus the longest overall diameter of any other intrahepatic or extrahepatic target lesions. Partial response (PR) is defined as a decrease of 30% or more in the sum diameter of the target lesions, taking as reference the baseline sum diameter. In contrast, progressive disease (PD) is defined as an increase of 20% or more in the sum diameter of the target lesions, taking as reference the smallest sum diameter of the target lesions recorded since treatment started. Stable disease (SD) is any case that shows neither sufficient decrease to qualify for PR nor sufficient increase to qualify for PD. Finally, complete response (CR) is a sum diameter of the target lesions of zero, that means the disappearance of any arterial enhancement in intrahepatic target lesions with typical vascular profile at baseline, plus the disappearance of any other intrahepatic or extrahepatic target lesions.

Of note, when measuring the viable (enhancing) portion of the tumors, reduced arterial perfusion due to changes in contrast injection protocol or local hemodynamics must be distinguished from actual necrosis. According to mRECIST, only tumors or tumor areas that show complete absence of any contrast uptake can be assumed to represent necrotic tissue. Quantitative determinations of contrast uptake obtained by comparing relevant regions of interest measurements on pre-contrast and post-contrast scans can be used, whenever considered appropriate, to support the subjective assessment.

Tumor necrosis should also be taken into account when assessing the response of non-target lesions. In particular, the CR of non-target lesions can be declared in front of the disappearance of any arterial enhancement in intrahepatic non-target lesions with typical vascular profile at baseline, plus the disappearance of any other intrahepatic or extrahepatic non-target lesions.

In mRECIST, similar to standard RECIST, the appearance of one or more new lesions declares PD regardless of the response achieved in target and non-target lesions. Therefore, it is of utmost importance to prevent overcalls of progression due to newly detected nodules erroneously classified as newly developed HCC tumors. In this regard, mRECIST provides strict recommendations for the classification of newly detected focal liver lesions as new HCC, based on the well-established criteria for the diagnosis of HCC in cirrhosis. Thus, a new liver lesion can be classified as HCC—and therefore considered as unequivocal evidence of progression—only when its longest diameter is at least 1 cm and the nodule shows hypervascularization in the arterial phase with washout in the portal venous or the late phase at CT or MRI. Any new liver lesion that is smaller than 1 cm or fails to show such typical enhancement profile should be considered as equivocal. Such lesions without typical vascular profile can be diagnosed as HCC by evidence of either a change in enhancement pattern or at least 1-cm interval growth in subsequent scans. To prevent artificial prolongation of time-to-progression (TTP), the mRECIST guideline also states that any individual radiological event can be adjudicated in retrospect as PD at the time it was first detected by imaging techniques, even if strict criteria were fulfilled only on subsequent radiological testing [7].

Of importance, these strict criteria for the diagnosis of new HCC lesions are not only important to avoid misdiagnoses of benign abnormalities or pseudolesions as HCC. They can actually prevent overcalls of progression due to HCC lesions that were present at baseline, but were undetectable because of the small size and/or the atypical vascular profile. In fact, such undetectable lesions may become visible on post-baseline imaging assessments due to the development of internal necrosis induced by the treatment. The development of internal necrosis results in a substantial increase in the difference in density between the focal lesion and the surrounding liver, "unmasking" the lesion itself and mimicking the emergence of a new lesion. The "appearance" of such a lesion on post-baseline assessments would be classified as progression according to standard RECIST, but does not lead to erroneous interpretations in mRECIST because the necrotic lesion will not meet the criteria to be classified as new HCC (Fig. 1).

For extrahepatic lesions, any lesion that is detected at a given post-baseline timepoint, is unequivocally malignant, and has no corresponding lesion on the baseline imaging will be considered as evidence of PD.

Assessment of Response to Loco-Regional Therapies

Several clinical investigations have shown that the tumor response measured by mRECIST predicts survival in patients receiving loco-regional therapies [10–18]. A recent meta-analysis identified seven clinical trials assessing survival outcomes after loco-regional treatments according to mRECIST response [19]. Each individual study showed better survival for responders (CR or PR) compared to non-responders (SD or PD). Overall, the meta-analysis included 1,357 patients. The hazard ratio for overall survival (responders versus non responders) was 0.39 (95% confidence interval 0.26–0.61, $p < 0.0001$) (Fig. 2).

An important issue to consider when evaluating the tumor response to loco-regional therapies, particularly transcatheter arterial chemoembolization (TACE), is the timepoint of the response assessment. It has been shown that a second TACE can induce objective response in nearly half of the patients who failed to achieve an

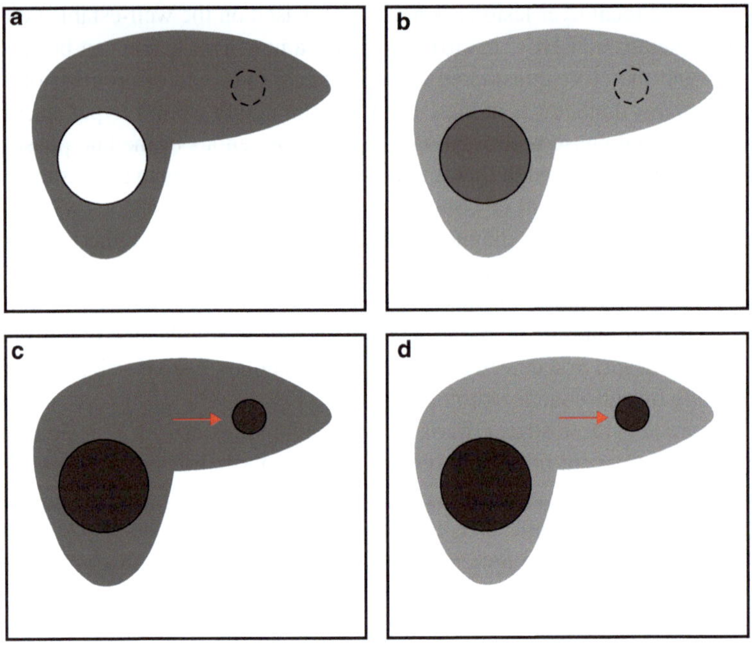

Fig. 1 Simulated example of a lesion unmasked by the development of internal necrosis induced by the treatment. Baseline arterial phase (**a**) and portal venous phase (**b**) scans identify the large lesion in the right lobe but fails to detect the lesion in the left lobe due to its small size and modest vascularity. The subject responds to treatment and both tumors develop massive internal necrosis. At the post-baseline assessment, the large lesion in the right lobe fails to show any enhancement in both the arterial (**c**) and the portal venous phase, meeting the criteria for complete response (**d**). The small lesion in the left lobe is unmasked and becomes detectable, mimicking the emergence of a new lesion. Contrary to standard RECIST, this finding does not lead to an erroneous classification of progression because the lesion does not meet the criteria to be classified as new HCC

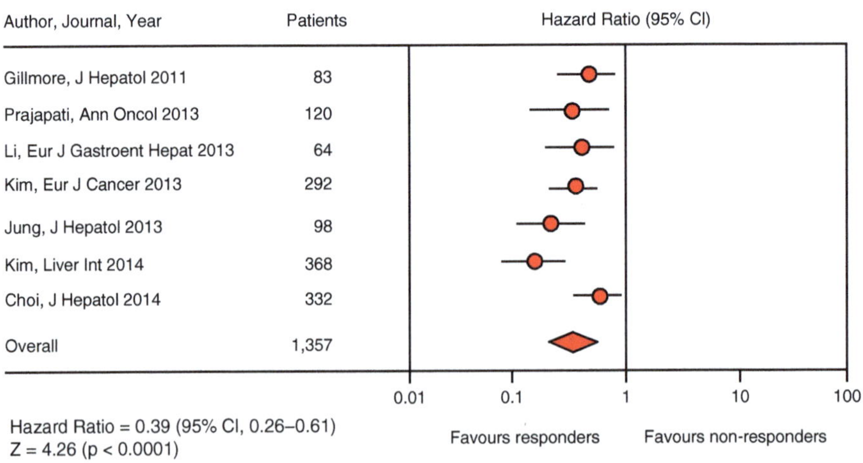

Fig. 2 Forest plot of hazard ratio for overall survival (responders vs non responders according to mRECIST) in patients receiving loco-regional treatment for HCC (adapted from [6]). *CI* confidence interval

objective response after the initial TACE [20]. Even in patients who show tumor progression during post-TACE follow-up, repeat TACE can achieve again a response, such as in the case of patients who develop a new intrahepatic nodule remote from the territory previously treated with TACE. Therefore, tumor progression after TACE is not synonymous of treatment failure and should not result in TACE discontinuation if the patient may still derive benefit from repeat TACE [21, 22].

Some other points deserve proper consideration. First, CR after loco-regional therapy is not synonymous of complete tumor eradication. Studies that evaluated imaging-pathology correlation have shown that residual viable tumor foci may be undetectable by imaging, although either complete or nearly complete necrosis is observed in most instances [23]. Unfortunately, this limitation is inherent in any imaging-based criteria. Second, while mRECIST has generally shown high intra-observer and inter-observer reproducibility, measurements of viable tumor diameters may be exposed to variability in lesions with heterogeneous distribution of the viable tumor tissue [24]. Image interpretation can be especially challenging after TACE with Lipiodol, although this limitation only affects CT and not MRI [25]. Third, the mechanism of action and time-dependence of the different forms of loco-regional interventions may be relevant to the timelines of the assessment, especially for treatments such as Yttrium-90 radioembolization that require time for response to manifest and may not lead to pronounced necrotic features.

Assessment of Response to Molecular Targeted Therapies

A limited number of retrospective studies investigated whether response assessment according to mRECIST predicts survival in patients treated with sorafenib. These studies consistently showed that patients who achieved objective response had a longer survival than non-responders [26–29]. Recently, Lencioni et al. [30] and Meyer et al. [31] confirmed that objective response by mRECIST predicts survival by using data from double blind randomized trials. The first study used data from the phase 3 study comparing brivanib versus placebo in second line [32]. In this trial, 210/226 (93%) patients in the brivanib arm and 101/108 (94%) in the placebo arm, who had baseline and on-study scans available for central blinded review, were evaluable according to mRECIST. An objective response was shown in 26/210 patients on brivanib and in 2/101 on placebo ($p < 0.01$). Median survival was 16.4 months (95% CI, 15.7–NA) for brivanib responders and 8.3 months (95% CI, 7.2–9.7) for brivanib non-responders (hazard ratio, 0.28; 95% CI, 0.14–0.55, $p < 0.01$), and mRECIST response was confirmed as an independent predictor of survival at multivariate time-dependent analysis [30]. The second study assessed data from two phase 2 trials conducted to evaluate the efficacy/safety of nintedanib versus sorafenib as first-line treatment of mainly Caucasian patients (NCT01004003) or Asian patients (NCT00987935) with advanced HCC. Data from 188 patients treated with either nintedanib or sorafenib were pooled for analyses. Response rates were 4.3% by standard RECIST and 14.9% by mRECIST. Overall survival was significantly longer in patients with response compared to patients without response; RECIST: HR 0.32 (95% CI 0.13–0.81), p = 0.01; mRECIST: 0.53 (95% CI 0.33–0.85), p = 0.008. RECIST response and mRECIST response were both significant predictors of survival at multivariate analysis, however mRECIST was able to identify 3 times more responders [32]. Both these clinical investigations concluded that objective mRECIST response is a surrogate for overall survival and as such should be considered a valid endpoint for use in HCC trials.

Several issues remain open. The reported percentages of sorafenib responders did not exceed 10–20%, with the majority of the patients showing limited changes in target lesions and, therefore, only qualifying for stable disease. While this is a major improvement with respect to the 2–3% response rate reported for standard RECIST in the SHARP and Asia-Pacific trials, it may not address the need to identify the maximum number of patients who benefit from the treatment. In fact, the threshold of a 30% reduction in diameter required by mRECIST to declare a PR has not been modified from the standard RECIST. Such a cut-off was used in the original RECIST model because it is the unidimensional equivalent of the bidimensional 50% reduction in the product of the longest perpendicular diameters that was adopted by the World Health Organization (WHO) in the very first definition of objective response, published in the 1979 WHO Handbook. Novel, non-dichotomous approaches to imaging assessment of tumor response have already been investigated, including the use of waterfall plots and kinetics measures of tumor size changes. While these approaches are still exploratory, efforts to develop and validate them as potential endpoints should be encouraged (Fig. 3).

Another emerging concept is that the pattern of tumor progression may have major implications for post-progression survival prediction. While the development of vascular invasion and extrahepatic spread have long been recognized as predictors of poor survival outcomes in patients treated by surgical or loco-regional therapies, recent work has shown that the pattern of tumor progression may also be relevant in patients with advanced disease receiving systemic therapy. In particular, it has been shown that survival after progression is significantly worse for patients who develop a new extrahepatic lesion and/or vascular invasion with respect to those who progress because of the growth of existing intrahepatic or extrahepatic lesions or because of the development of a new intrahepatic lesion [33, 34]. The mRECIST model already captures the different patterns of progression. However, specific case report forms or other data collection methods may be needed to facilitate subsequent calculations of endpoints such as TTP according to the subclass of progression.

Assessment of Response to Immuno-Therapies

With the advent of immune checkpoint inhibitors, the basic structure of the RECIST model might require substantial changes. As shown in the setting of melanoma patients treated with immunotherapies, the standard RECIST may not provide a reliable assessment of the antitumor effect [35]. In fact, the response to immunotherapy

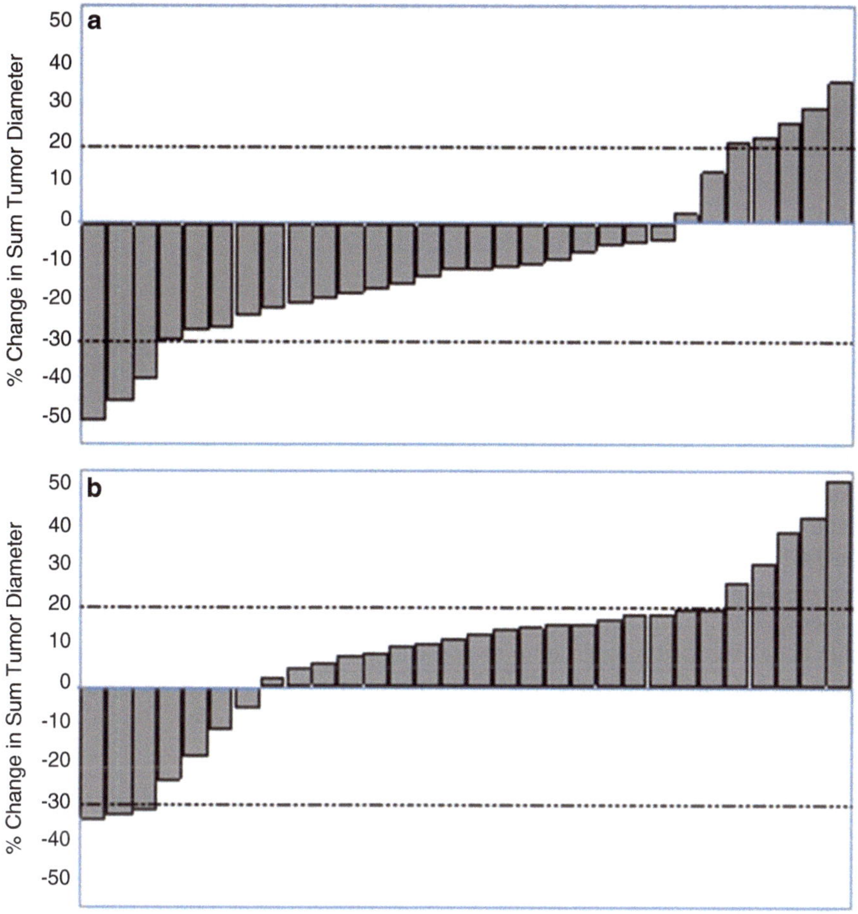

Fig. 3 Simulated examples of waterfall plots depicting the percentage change in tumor burden, as evidenced by the sum diameter of the target lesions. The agent depicted in (**a**) appears to have higher antitumor activity than the agent depicted in (**b**), although the number of subjects who qualify for objective response or progressive disease is actually identical in both panels

may take longer compared to other agents, and can manifest after imaging features that meet the current criteria for progression. In particular, two "pseudoprogression" patterns have been described: (a) response that occurs after an initial increase in total tumor burden; and (b) response that occurs during or after the appearance of new lesions [36].

Immune-related response criteria have been developed, that address these issues by including a "confirmation of progression" by a second scan obtained at least 4 weeks after progressive disease has been registered (similar to the concept of confirmed response) and incorporate new lesions into "total tumor burden" by summing their diameter to the diameter of the target lesions. With this conceptual change in the assessment of new lesions, patients are considered to have objective response or stable disease even if new lesions are present, as long as they meet the respective thresholds. Furthermore, patients are not considered to have progressive disease if new lesions are present but the tumor burden of all lesions does not increase above the threshold for progression. Investigation of these approaches in the setting of HCC clinical trials is clearly a top priority.

Conclusions

Assessment of HCC response to treatment entails unique complexities and requires adequate background and skills for proper image interpretation. The mRECIST model was implemented 7 years ago and since then has been used at a level far beyond expectation. Differences in response categories registered by mRECIST appear to reflect real biologic changes in the tumor with clinically meaningful implications. Of importance, mRECIST criteria by themselves do not declare what parameters should signal that a new agent has activity worth pursuing further. The mRECIST model simply describes how to collect and categorize objective observations of tumor changes over time and offers a framework to investigate novel potential endpoints that are supposed to be a better surrogate for survival. Finally, caution should be exercised in translating response assessment models developed for clinical trials into clinical practice. The evaluation of tumor response in the daily clinical practice may be based on a subjective medical judgment that results from a comprehensive assessment of all clinical, imaging, and laboratory data.

Conflict of Interest Nothing to declare.

References

1. Therasse P, Arbuck SG, Eisenhauer EA, et al. New guidelines to evaluate the response to treatment in solid tumors. J Natl Cancer Inst. 2000;92:205–16.
2. Eisenhauer EA, Therasse P, Bogaerts J, et al. New response evaluation criteria in solid tumours: revised RECIST guideline (version 1.1). Eur J Cancer. 2009;45:228–47.
3. Llovet JM, Ricci S, Mazzaferro V, et al. Sorafenib in advanced hepatocellular carcinoma. N Engl J Med. 2008;359:378–90.
4. Cheng AL, Kang YK, Chen Z, et al. Efficacy and safety of sorafenib in patients in the Asia-Pacific region with advanced hepatocellular carcinoma: a phase III randomised, double-blind, placebo-controlled trial. Lancet Oncol. 2009;10:25–34.
5. Kane RC, Farrell AT, Madabushi R, et al. Sorafenib for the treatment of unresectable hepatocellular carcinoma. Oncologist. 2009;14:95–100.
6. Llovet JM, Di Bisceglie AM, Bruix J, et al. Panel of Experts in HCC Clinical Trials. Design and endpoints of clinical trials in hepatocellular carcinoma. J Natl Cancer Inst. 2008;100:698–711.
7. Lencioni R, Llovet JM. Modified RECIST (mRECIST) assessment for hepatocellular carcinoma. Semin Liver Dis. 2010;30:52–60.
8. Verslype C, Rosmorduc O, Rougier P, ESMO Guidelines Working Group. Hepatocellular carcinoma: ESMO-ESDO clinical practice guidelines for diagnosis, treatment and follow-up. Ann Oncol. 2012;23(Suppl 7):vii41–8.

9. European Association for the Study of the Liver; European Organisation for Research and Treatment of Cancer. EASL-EORTC clinical practice guidelines: management of hepatocellular carcinoma. J Hepatol. 2012;56:908–43.
10. Gillmore R, Stuart S, Kirkwood A, Hameeduddin A, Woodward N, Burroughs AK, Meyer T. EASL and mRECIST responses are independent prognostic factors for survival in hepatocellular cancer patients treated with transarterial embolisation. J Hepatol. 2011;55:1309–16.
11. Shim JH, Lee HC, Kim SO, Shin YM, Kim KM, Lim YS, Suh DJ. Which response criteria best help predict survival of patients with hepatocellular carcinoma following chemoembolization? A validation study of old and new models. Radiology. 2012;262:708–18.
12. Prajapati HJ, Spivey JR, Hanish SI, El-Rayes BF, Kauh JS, Chen Z, Kim HS. mRECIST and EASL responses at early time point by contrast-enhanced dynamic MRI predict survival in patients with unresectable hepatocellular carcinoma (HCC) treated by doxorubicin drug-eluting beads transarterial chemoembolization (DEB TACE). Ann Oncol. 2013;24:965–73.
13. Shim JH, Han S, Shin YM, et al. Optimal measurement modality and method for evaluation of responses to transarterial chemoembolization of hepatocellular carcinoma based on enhancement criteria. J Vasc Interv Radiol. 2013;24:316–25.
14. Yeo DM, Choi JI, Lee YJ, Park MY, Chun HJ, Lee HG. Comparison of RECIST, mRECIST, and choi criteria for early response evaluation of hepatocellular carcinoma after transarterial chemoembolization using drug-eluting beads. J Comput Assist Tomogr. 2014;38:391–7.
15. Hyun D, Shin SW, Cho SK, et al. Efficacy of RECIST and mRECIST criteria as prognostic factors in patients undergoing repeated iodized oil chemoembolization of intermediate stage hepatocellular carcinoma. Acta Radiol. 2015;56:1437–45.
16. Ichikawa T, Machida N, Sasaki H, et al. Early prediction of the outcome using tumor markers and mRECIST in unresectable hepatocellular carcinoma patients who underwent transarterial chemoembolization. Oncology. 2016;91:317–30.
17. Mosconi C, Gramenzi A, Ascanio S, et al. Yttrium-90 radioembolization for unresectable/recurrent intrahepatic cholangiocarcinoma: a survival, efficacy and safety study. Br J Cancer. 2016;115:297–302.
18. Lencioni R. New data supporting modified RECIST (mRECIST) for hepatocellular carcinoma. Clin Cancer Res. 2013;19:1312–4.
19. Vincenzi B, Di Maio M, Silletta M, et al. Prognostic relevance of objective response according to EASL criteria and mRECIST criteria in hepatocellular carcinoma patients treated with loco-regional therapies: a literature-based meta-analysis. PLoS One. 2015;10:e0133488.
20. Georgiades C, Geschwind JF, Harrison N, et al. Lack of response after initial chemoembolization for hepatocellular carcinoma: does it predict failure of subsequent treatment? Radiology. 2012;265:115–23.
21. Bruix J, Reig M, Rimola J, et al. Clinical decision making and research in hepatocellular carcinoma: pivotal role of imaging techniques. Hepatology. 2011;54:2238–44.
22. Lencioni R, Llovet JM, Han G, et al. Sorafenib or placebo plus TACE with doxorubicin-eluting beads for intermediate-stage HCC: the SPACE trial. J Hepatol. 2016;64:1090–8.
23. Bargellini I, Bozzi E, Campani D, et al. Modified RECIST to assess tumor response after transarterial chemoembolization of hepatocellular carcinoma: CT-pathologic correlation in 178 liver explants. Eur J Radiol. 2013;82:e212–8.
24. Seyal AR, Gonzalez-Guindalini FD, Arslanoglu A, et al. Reproducibility of mRECIST in assessing response to transarterial radioembolization therapy in hepatocellular carcinoma. Hepatology. 2015;62:1111–21.
25. Lencioni R, de Baere T, Soulen MC, Rilling WS, Geschwind JH. Lipiodol transarterial chemoembolization for hepatocellular carcinoma: a systematic review of efficacy and safety data. Hepatology. 2016;64:106–16.
26. Edeline J, Boucher E, Rolland Y, et al. Comparison of tumor response by Response Evaluation Criteria in Solid Tumors (RECIST) and modified RECIST in patients treated with sorafenib for hepatocellular carcinoma. Cancer. 2012;118:147–56.
27. Ronot M, Bouattour M, Wassermann J, et al. Alternative response criteria (Choi, European association for the study of the liver, and modified Response Evaluation Criteria in Solid

Tumors [RECIST]) versus RECIST 1.1 in patients with advanced hepatocellular carcinoma treated with sorafenib. Oncologist. 2014;19:394–402.
28. Takada J, Hidaka H, Nakazawa T, et al. Modified response evaluation criteria in solid tumors is superior to response evaluation criteria in solid tumors for assessment of responses to sorafenib in patients with advanced hepatocellular carcinoma. BMC Res Notes. 2015;8:609.
29. Wang W, Bai W, Wang E, et al. mRECIST response combined with sorafenib-related adverse events is superior to either criterion alone in predicting survival in HCC patients treated with TACE plus sorafenib. Int J Cancer. 2016;140(2):390–9. [Epub ahead of print]
30. Lencioni R, Montal R, Torres F, et al. Objective response by mRECIST as a predictor and potential surrogate endpoint of overall survival in advanced HCC. J Hepatol. 2017.; [Epub ahead of print]
31. Meyer T, Palmer DH, Cheng AL, et al. mRECIST to predict survival in advanced HCC: analysis of two randomised phase II trials comparing nintedanib versus sorafenib. Liver Int. 2017.; [Epub ahead of print]
32. Llovet JM, Decaens T, Raoul JL, et al. Brivanib in patients with advanced hepatocellular carcinoma who were intolerant to sorafenib or for whom sorafenib failed: results from the randomized phase III BRISK-PS study. J Clin Oncol. 2013;31:3509–16.
33. Reig M, Rimola J, Torres F, et al. Postprogression survival of patients with advanced hepatocellular carcinoma: rationale for second-line trial design. Hepatology. 2013;58:2023–31.
34. Iavarone M, Cabibbo G, Biolato M, et al. Predictors of survival in patients with advanced hepatocellular carcinoma who permanently discontinued sorafenib. Hepatology. 2015;62:784–91.
35. Hodi FS, Hwu WJ, Kefford R, et al. Evaluation of immune-related response criteria and RECIST v1.1 in patients with advanced melanoma treated with pembrolizumab. J Clin Oncol. 2016;34:1510–7.
36. Wolchok JD, Hoos A, O'Day S, et al. Guidelines for the evaluation of immune therapy activity in solid tumors: immune-related response criteria. Clin Cancer Res. 2009;15:7412–20.

Sorafenib and Clinical Patterns of Resistance in Hepatocellular Carcinoma

Maria Reig, Álvaro Díaz-Gonzalez, Andrea Ribeiro, and Anna Darnell

Abstract Sorafenib is the first-line systemic treatment in hepatocellular carcinoma (HCC). The benefits of sorafenib in HCC show an improvement in overall survival and delay of radiologic tumor progression. These benefits were demonstrated in the absence of a high rate of overall response and the magnitude of this improvement varies considerably from patient to patient. Several hypotheses have tried to address the reason for this variability, giving birth to the emerging field of sorafenib resistance. The aim of this chapter is to discuss the clinical evolutionary events such as early dermatologic adverse events, pattern of progression or serum biomarkers modification that have an impact both on the patient's outcome as well as in the patient's management. The pattern of progression classifies patients in four different groups: (1) intra-hepatic (2) extra-hepatic increase in tumor size (3) new intra-hepatic lesion and (4) new extra-hepatic lesion and it is correlated with the post-progression overall survival. Hence, careful evaluation of patients characteristics and their evolutionary events during sorafenib treatment are key to identify the best candidates to continue on sorafenib, those who should receive regorafenib as second-line treatment, second-line trials or best supportive care. In addition, the design of second- and third-line clinical trials should consider all the components discussed in this chapter.

Keywords Hepatocellular carcinoma • Sorafenib • Resistance • Overall survival • Adverse events • Pattern of progression • Post-progression survival

---

M. Reig (✉) • Á. Díaz-Gonzalez • A. Ribeiro
Barcelona Clinic Liver Cancer (BCLC) Group, Liver Unit, Hospital Clinic Barcelona, IDIBAPS, University of Barcelona, Barcelona, Spain

Centro de Investigación Biomédica en Red de Enfermedades Hepáticas y Digestivas (CIBERehd), c/Villarroel, 170. Escala 11, 4ª planta, 08036 Barcelona, Spain
e-mail: mreig1@clinic.ub.es

A. Darnell
Department of Radiology, BCLC Group, Hospital Clinic Barcelona, University of Barcelona, Barcelona, Spain

A. Villanueva (ed.), *Resistance to Molecular Therapies for Hepatocellular Carcinoma*, Resistance to Targeted Anti-Cancer Therapeutics,
DOI 10.1007/978-3-319-56197-4_7

Abbreviations

AE	Adverse event
AFP	Alpha-fetoprotein
ANGPT2	Angiopoyetin-2
BCLC	Barcelona Clinic Liver Cancer
DAE60	DAEs within the first 60 days requiring sorafenib dose modification
DAEs	Dermatologic adverse events
EASL	European Association for the Study of Liver Diseases
HCC	Hepatocellular carcinoma
HGF	Hepatocyte growth factor
PDGFR-β	Platelet-derived growth factor receptor β
PPS	Post-progression survival
TTP	Time to progression
VEGFRs	Vascular endothelial growth factor receptor

Introduction

Sorafenib is the first line systemic treatment in hepatocellular carcinoma (HCC). It is a small molecule that inhibits tumor cell proliferation and tumor angiogenesis, and increases the rate of apoptosis by inhibiting the activity of BRAF and the vascular endothelial growth factor receptors (VEGFRs) 1, 2, and 3 as well as the platelet-derived growth factor receptor β (PDGFR-β) [1].

The benefits of sorafenib in HCC were demonstrated in 2007 (i.e., the SHARP trial [2] -Phase III, randomized sorafenib versus placebo- and also in the Asian-Pacific trial [3]) showing an improvement in overall survival (HR = 0.69; 95% confidence interval, 0.55–0.87; $P < 0.001$) and delay of radiologic tumor progression (HR = 0.58; 95% confidence interval, 0.45–0.74) [2]. These benefits were demonstrated in the absence of a high rate of overall response but with a good safety profile. The survival benefit of sorafenib is maintained regardless of the patients' baseline characteristics [4], but the magnitude of this improvement varies considerably. This variability is also evident when stratifying the patients according to homogeneous baseline characteristics such as tumor burden (stages BCLC-C or BCLC-B [5–7]), liver function (Child-Pugh score A/B [5, 6, 8, 9]) or performance status (0/1 [6, 9, 10]).

Thus, a great effort has been made to understand the mechanisms of action of sorafenib and its impact on patient outcome. However, the intensity of how the drug inhibits its different targets is heterogeneous, and hence, the specific effect responsible for the survival benefit is still unknown. Several hypotheses have tried to address this issue, giving birth to the emerging field of sorafenib resistance and how it could potentially help understand the differences found in patients outcomes [11].

Nevertheless, how do we define 'sorafenib resistance'? Is it necessary to talk about 'sorafenib resistance'? In other words, do we need to include in this equation the role of known prognostic factors to better understand the patients' evolution before considering that they have failed to respond to sorafenib due to intolerance or progression?

The aim of this chapter is to discuss the clinical evolutionary events that have an impact both on the patient outcome as well as in the patient management [12]. In addition, it will underscore the need to differentiate the inappropriate use of terminology such as 'resistance' to clinical situations related to an inappropriate indication of the drug.

To define the clinical patterns of outcome in HCC patients treated with sorafenib, the integration of the already known baseline prognostic factors defined in the BCLC-stage and the evolutionary events that emerge during sorafenib treatment (e.g., adverse events, radiological responses, cirrhosis complications, alpha-fetoprotein (AFP) dynamics and other confounding factors) are required.

Adverse Events in HCC Patients Receiving Sorafenib

In the SHARP trial [2], 80% of the patients presented at least one adverse event (AE) of any grade. The percentage of any grade of AEs was significantly different in the sorafenib arm compared to placebo, but the percentage of severe AEs was similar in both arms. HCC patients under sorafenib treatment may develop cirrhosis complications, sorafenib-related AEs such as dermatologic reactions (Fig. 1), diarrhea, hypophosphatemia or non sorafenib-related AEs. Thus, even more complex than 'sorafenib-resistance' is the definition of 'sorafenib-tolerance', which is sometimes based on the minimal dose that the patient receives. For this reason, the direct

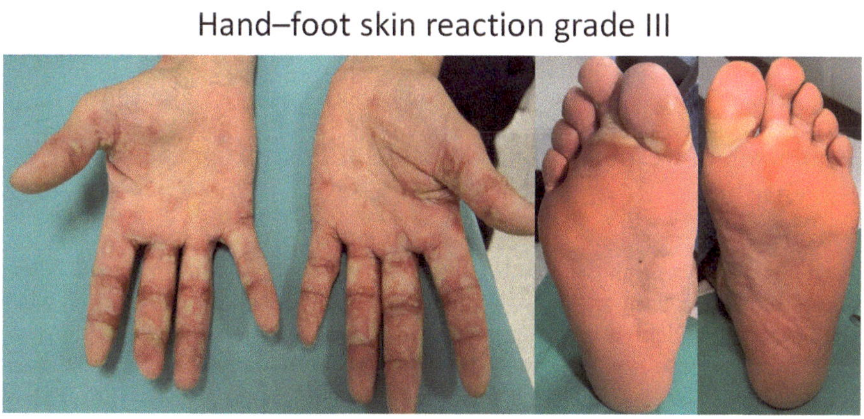

Fig. 1 Dermatologic skin reaction grade III

association of 'sorafenib-intolerance' with 'sorafenib-resistance' is a misinterpretation of the issue. The impossibility of receiving the drug due to intolerance is not the same as not obtaining its benefits. Hence, it order to understand the mechanism of resistance to sorafenib, it is critical to accurate discriminate between these clinical scenarios. The best example of this conflicting situation is the development of dermatologic adverse events (DAEs) in patients who are treated with sorafenib [13–18]. Historically, adverse events were seen as a negative point in the management of cancer patients treated with systemic treatment [19–21]. However, retrospective analyses showed how DAEs were associated with better overall survival than patients who did not develop any dermatological toxicity [13–15]. In addition, our prospective study in which the DAEs were considered evolutionary events and time-dependent analysis was applied, patients who developed DAEs within the first 60 days and needed sorafenib dose modification (DAE60) presented better survival and time to progression (TTP) than those who did not develop DAE or who developed mild dermatologic reactions without the need to modify sorafenib [17]. Branco et al. also validated this association in an external cohort [18]. Thus, the direct association of 'intolerance' with 'resistance' induces a bias in the prediction of patient evolution. Indeed, patients who developed DAE60 and continued on sorafenib with less than half dose represent the majority of the patients who achieved complete response in a multicentre study with more than 1,000 patients which was done in Spain [22]. This association allows us to speculate a potential association between hypoxia and immuno/inflammatory reaction [23] in patients who are treated with sorafenib. Nevertheless, the mechanism involved in the development of HCC radiologic response, tumor progression or adverse events is still unclear. Thus, the impact of hypoxia on the tumor microenvironment and/or the development of adverse events need to be considered [24, 25].

In line with this, a recent publication by Ponziani et al. [26] showed better overall survival in patients who developed relevant AE, defined as higher than grade 2, than those who presented minor AE. Therefore, sorafenib dose adjustments are essential before considering sorafenib-intolerance in clinical practice due to the impact of relevant AE on patient survival. The impact of other AEs on survival was also evaluated but additional data are still needed to adequately assess its true significance.

Radiological Responses and the Role of Post-progression Survival

Radiologic tumor progression was considered synonymous with treatment failure and/or indirect criteria of drug resistance [27, 28]. This belief was dispelled when the SHARP trial demonstrated an improvement on overall survival, with a low rate of overall response (i.e., 2% and 1% in the sorafenib and placebo arms, respectively) [2] but associated with a delay of radiologic tumor progression (i.e., TTP of 5.5 and 2.8 months in sorafenib and placebo arms, respectively) [2, 29].

Thus, since 2008 many authors have tried to improve the quality of the radiologic response assessment in systemic treatment and have developed new criteria or modified the previous criteria [30–33]. The aim of all these criteria is to better identify patients who achieve objective response and divide them into 'responder vs. non-responder', even despite sorafenib delays tumor progression but does not achieve objective response. Hence, the main difference between the criteria is based on the proportion of patients who are classified as having 'stable disease' or 'partial response'. Nevertheless, the proportion of patients with tumor progression according to EASL [34], RECIST 1.1 [28], modified-RECIST [30] and Choi [31] criteria is similar regardless of the criteria used when compared within the same cohort [32, 33]. Unfortunately, none of the 'new criteria' have been compared with the radiologic criteria used in the SHARP trial (BCLC-RECIST) [29]. Consequently, the question now is how do we define resistance in HCC patients treated with sorafenib? Is radiologic progression enough to define resistance [35]? Another chapter in this book will focus on the role of radiology evaluation in HCC patients.

It is already known that tumor progression is a poor prognostic factor in HCC patients but this issue is not strong enough to correctly characterize the patients' post-progression survival (PPS) [5, 35]. Post-progression survival can be defined as the time between when radiologic tumor progression is identified and the patient dies or last follow-up. PPS depends on three factors: (1) underlying liver function, (2) tumor-related symptoms, and (3) pattern of radiologic tumor progression [5, 36, 37]. The first two are universally known but the third one was described for the first time in 2013 [5]. Thus, the pattern of progression classifies patients in four different groups: (1) intra-hepatic or (2) extra-hepatic increase in tumor size, (3) new intra-hepatic lesion, and (4) new extra-hepatic lesion.

The impact of pattern of progression on post-progression survival (PPS) was evaluated in 147 HCC patients (HCV 57%, PS-0 84%, Child–Pugh A 82% and 52% BCLC-B with failure or contraindications to surgery or loco-regional treatment). The following variables were identified as independent predictors of overall survival in the whole cohort: baseline BCLC ($p < 0.001$), performance status (PS, $p = 0.02$), Child-Pugh score modification ($p < 0.001$), definitive interruption of sorafenib ($p < 0.0001$) and time to tumor progression ($p < 0.001$). However, the presence of a new extra-hepatic lesion ($p = 0.004$) was also an independent predictor of overall and post-progression survival in patients with radiologic progression, preserved liver function and no or mild tumor related-symptoms [5]. This data has been further validated in an Italian [36] and Japanese cohorts [37].

Hence, we could consider three scenarios according to the radiological progression: (a) patients with radiologic tumor progression due to new extra-hepatic lesion, preserved liver function and mild-related symptoms (potential radiologic tumor resistance). This group of patients have the all the worse prognosis factors and is expected to have the worse post-progression survival; (b) patients with radiologic tumor progression due to other patterns of progression (intrahepatic/extrahepatic increase in tumor size, new intra-hepatic lesion), good liver function and without mild tumor-related symptoms (no radiological tumor resistance). Thus, intrahepatic/extrahepatic increase in tumor size and new intra-hepatic lesion patterns are

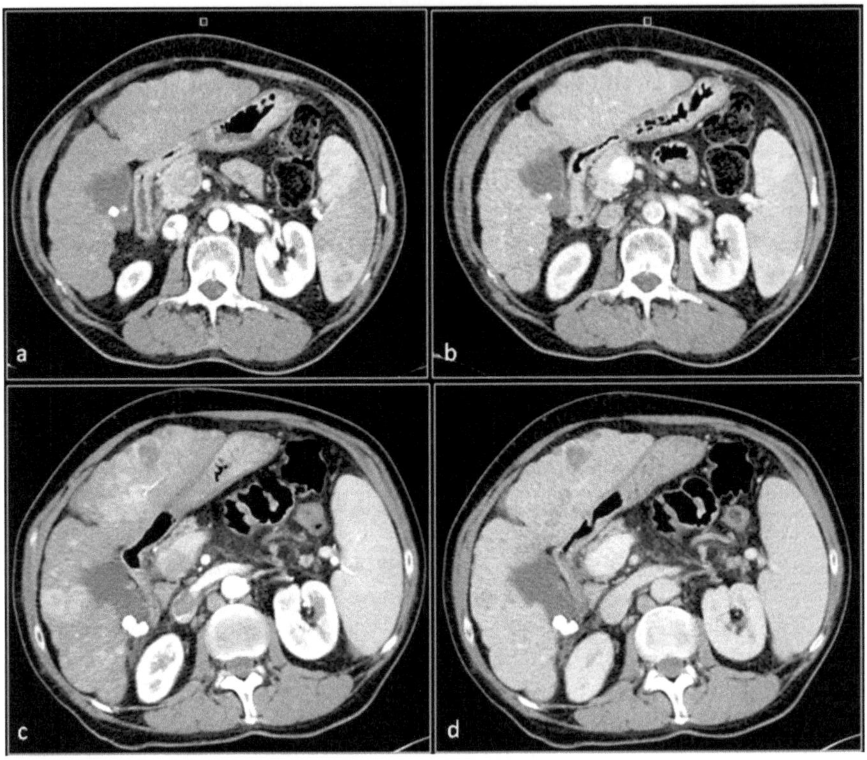

Fig. 2 (**a**) Arterial and (**b**) portal phase baseline CT scan. (**c**) Arterial and (**d**) portal phase CT 10 months after Sorafenib. Intrahepatic progression

not independent predictors of PPS (Fig. 2). This group should not be considered as treatment failure and their post-progression survival is between 14 and 24 months [5]; (c) HCC patients with radiologic tumor progression regardless of the pattern, liver dysfunction and/or tumor related-symptoms. These patients represent those with symptomatic progression.

Cirrhosis Complications as Confounders of Sorafenib Resistance

Patients on sorafenib are at risk of developing cirrhosis complications [38–40], but is it the development of a cirrhotic complication an indirect sign of sorafenib resistance? It is important to distinguish if a given clinical event represents a complication of cirrhosis that could appear independently of sorafenib, a consequence of tumor progression [41, 42], or if it is an AE potentially related to the drug. If the event requires for sorafenib to be interrupted, the decision to re-start treatment will depend on this distinction. For example, if a patient presents a liver dysfunction defined by an increase on his Child-Pugh score, this could be due to an increase of bilirubin, a decrease of albumin or prothrombin time, or to the development of ascites or encephalopathy. In most instances, these events translate liver function impairment. However, they could sometimes be a consequence of other confounding factors, which are not primarily related to liver dysfunction [12]. For instance, an increase of indirect bilirubin may be due to the interaction of sorafenib with bilirubin metabolism [43, 44]. Also, a decrease in prothrombin time may be due to concomitant medication (e.g., warfarin). Encephalopathy may be precipitated by drug related constipation, which is easily resolved [45]. Thus, a critical analysis of these aspects is mandatory before considering a clinical event as a clear sign of sorafenib resistance.

The Role of Alpha-Fetoprotein (AFP) Evolution as a Marker of Resistance

AFP is a well know HCC prognostic factor, but its determination is not recommended for screening and/or diagnosis due to its low overall accuracy in this clinical scenario [46, 47]. Even more important, it has not been used in clinical practice to predict treatment evolution or define sorafenib-resistance [46, 47]. Once again, many questions arise regarding the use of AFP to define: how do we define resistance according to AFP levels [11]? How many measurements are needed prior a definitive diagnosis of resistance? If we do not have a second determination due to early tumor progression or intolerance to sorafenib, should this patient still be considered as resistant? How do we define resistance in patients with normal baseline AFP? Some of these questions were raised some years ago, and Table 1 summarizes the articles [4, 48–58], which focused on AFP as a tool to predict the evolution of HCC patients treated by non-loco-regional therapies or resection.

Nevertheless, the main limitation of analyzing AFP levels in HCC patients is their unpredictable fluctuation and the need to analyze them with time-dependent analysis such as an evolutionary event (which was not done in the published data). In addition, Table 1 reflects the percentage of patients who were excluded from the analysis due to normal levels at baseline or due to early discontinuation.

Other Potential Confounding Factors When Defining Sorafenib Resistance

The pharmacokinetics of sorafenib [59–61] and pharmacogenomic profile [62] of the patient could also impact HCC evolution on an individual basis. However, up to now, measurement of sorafenib levels is not part of the clinical practice, nor the study of any specific patient haplotype.

Table 1 Summary of the articles that evaluated AFP as a tool to predict the evolution of HCC patients treated by non-loco-regional treatment or resection

				Patients N (%)		AFP					
						Responder criteria	Exclusion criteria due to AFP value		Exclusion criteria early discontinuation		Patient excluded for AFP analysis due to AFP criteria exclusion and/or early discontinuation
Author	Year	Drug	Type of study	Whole cohort	Analyzed patients	Criteria of AFP responder	Cut-off	% of excluded patient of the whole cohort	Due to adverse events (%)	Due to progression (%)	Total (%)
Cheng et al. [3]	2005	Thalidomide	Prospective	42	37 (88%)	Decrease of 50% or more	< 200 ng/mL	***Not reported***	2 (5%)	3 (7%)	10.0
Chan et al. [49]	2009	Doxorrubicin or PIAF (cisplatino plus IFN plus doxorrubicin and fluorouracil)	Retrospective	188	117 (62.2%)	Decrease of 20% or more	< 20 μg/L	***32 (17)***	28 (14.9)		31.9
Vora et al. [50]	2009	Gemcitabine, epirrubicine plus thalidomide, gecitabina/oxaliplatin plus bevacizumab, cetuximab or sunitinib	Retrospective	144	107 (74.3%)	Decrease of 50% or more	6.1–8.7 ng/mL	***18 (12.5)***	8 (7.5)		20
Shao et al. [51]	2010	Sorafenib plus tegafur/uracil, Bevacizumab plus capecitabine, thalidomide plus tegafur/uracil	Retrospective	107	72 (67.3%)	Decrease of 20% or more within the 1st month	< 20 ng/mL	***22 (20.6)***	3 (2.8)	11 (10.3)	33.7

Kuzuya et al. [52]	2011	Sorafenib	Prospective	52	39 (75%)	Ratio ≤ 1.2	Not reported	***Not reported***	Not reported		Not reported
Yau et al. [53]	2011	Sorafenib	Prospective	173	94 (54.3%)	Decrease of 20% or more	< 20 μg/L	***NA***			
			Exploration	51	41 (80.4%)			***10 (19.6)***	Not reported		21.6
			Validation	122	53 (43.4%)			***30 (24.6)***	26 (21.3)	Not reported	45.9
Raoul et al. [4]	2012	Sorafenib	Prospective/ retrospective	602	573 (95.2%)	Not elevated: 12.4 months. Mild elevation: 10.3 months. Moderate elevation: 7 months	Not reported	***29 (4.8)***	17 (2.8)[a]		7.6
Kawaoka et al. [54]	2012	Sorafenib	Retrospective	66	49 (74.2%)	AFP ratio ≤ 1 at week 8	NA	***No exclusion***	6 (9)	17(25.8)	34.8
Personeni et al. [55]	2012	Sorafenib from phase II Sorafenib, SHARP, phase II escalating Sorafenib vs Best Supportive Care	Retrospective	Not reported	85	Decrease of 20% or more	< 20 ng/ mL	***Not reported***	Not reported		Not reported

(continued)

Table 1 (continued)

Author	Year	Drug	Type of study	Patients N (%)		AFP					
						Responder criteria	Exclusion criteria due to AFP value		Exclusion criteria early discontinuation		Patient excluded for AFP analysis due to AFP criteria exclusion and/or early discontinuation
				Whole cohort	Analyzed patients	Criteria of AFP responder	Cut-off	% of excluded patient of the whole cohort	Due to adverse events (%)	Due to progression (%)	Total (%)
Nakazawa et al. [56]	2013	Sorafenib	Retrospective	59	57 (96.1%)	Increase ≤20%	< 10 ng/mL	***No exclusion***	Not reported	Yes (3.9%)	3.9
Varela et al. [57]	2014	Sorafenib	Prospective	114	83 (72.9%)	No increase of AFP above nadir on day 90	No increase in first 90 days	***33 (27.1)***	Not reported	Yes 7 (6.1%)	33.2
Kuzuya et al. [58]	2015	Soraenib	Prospective	123	57 (46.3%)	Ratio ≤ 1.2	< 20 ng/mL	***33 (26.8)***	Not reported		Not reported

AFP alpha-fetoprotein. Ratio (Kuzuya et al.): AFP from baseline to 2 and 4 weeks. *NA* not available. Ratio (Kawaoka et al.): Ratio AFP (week 8/baseline)
[a]The information it is not clear in the text

Serum biomarkers were evaluated in the context of the SHARP trial [2]. Despite VEGF and Ang-2 were identified as prognostic factors, none of the markers evaluated were able to predict response to sorafenib [63]. In this regard, some of the limitations of biomarkers are the absence of a pre-established normal value [63, 64], the wide spectrum of values according to each patient and the complexity in the interpretation of the results. Biomarker levels are likely to change in parallel to HCC evolution so time-dependent analysis as well as other confounding factors must be considered when analyzing the results [60]. For this reason, we have developed a prognostic score to improve the prediction of overall survival based on known prognostic factors and a novel set of serum biomarkers. The statistical analyses were done using both baseline characteristics and evolutionary events (i.e., time-dependent analysis). A set of serum biomarkers (i.e., angiopoyetin-2 (ANGPT2), VEGF, carbonic anhydrase IX [65], hepatocyte growth factor (HGF), CKIT and AFP) was measured at baseline, 1 and 3 months in 89 HCC patients treated with sorafenib. Their clinical characteristics included 54% HCV, 82% PS-0, 92% Child-Pugh-A and 48% BCLC-B. In addition, monthly clinical and laboratory work-up were performed, tumor progression was assessed at month 1 and every 2 months thereafter and the treatment was maintained until symptomatic progression, toxicity or inclusion of the patient in a second line clinical trial [66, 67].

We found that baseline levels of ANGPT2 and carbonic anhydrase IX and/or ANGPT2 as well as BCLC stage, PS, pattern of progression and the development of early dermatologic adverse events at month 1 were independent predictors of overall survival. Thus, when externally validated this score will become a very useful tool in clinical practice. It will surely improve the accuracy of survival prediction and help stratify patients at inclusion in second line clinical trials [67].

Fortunately, the RESORCE trial [68] (a multicenter, placebo-controlled phase III randomized clinical trial testing regorafenib in patients intolerant or who progressed to sorafenib) is the first positive second-line trial. Up to now, sorafenib was continued until the patient developed a symptomatic progression or he/she could be enrolled in a second line clinical trial. However, with the incorporation of regorafenib as a second-line treatment in HCC, this recommendation will likely change in the near future. As a result, a better characterization of resistance in patients under sorafenib will become paramount. Hence, careful evaluation of patient characteristics and their evolutionary events during sorafenib treatment are key to identify the best candidates to continue on sorafenib, those who should receive regorafenib as second line or be offered best supportive care. In addition, the design of second and third line clinical trials should consider all the components discussed in this chapter.

Conflict of Interest Maria Reig = Advisory boards, conferences, travel grants from Bayer.

References

1. Wilhelm SM, Carter C, Tang L, Wilkie D, McNabola A, Rong H, et al. BAY 43-9006 exhibits broad spectrum oral antitumor activity and targets the RAF/MEK/ERK pathway and receptor tyrosine kinases involved in tumor progression and angiogenesis. Cancer Res. 2004;64:7099–109.
2. Llovet JM, Ricci S, Mazzaferro V, Hilgard P, Gane E, Blanc JF, et al. Sorafenib in advanced hepatocellular carcinoma. N Engl J Med. 2008;359:378–90. doi:10.1056/NEJMoa0708857.
3. Cheng AL, Kang YK, Chen Z, Tsao CJ, Qin S, Kim JS, et al. Efficacy and safety of sorafenib in patients in the Asia-Pacific region with advanced hepatocellular carcinoma: a phase III randomised, double-blind, placebo-controlled trial. Lancet Oncol. 2009;10:25–34. doi:10.1016/S1470-2045(08)70285-7.
4. Raoul JL, Bruix J, Greten TF, Sherman M, Mazzaferro V, Hilgard P, et al. Relationship between baseline hepatic status and outcome, and effect of sorafenib on liver function: SHARP trial subanalyses. J Hepatol. 2012;56:1080–8. doi:10.1016/j.jhep.2011.12.009.
5. Reig M, Rimola J, Torres F, Darnell A, Rodriguez-Lope C, Forner A, et al. Postprogression survival of patients with advanced hepatocellular carcinoma: rationale for second-line trial design. Hepatology. 2013;58:2023–31. doi:10.1002/hep.26586.
6. Marrero JA, Kudo M, Venook AP, Ye S-L, Bronowicki J-P, Chen X-P, et al. Observational registry of sorafenib use in clinical practice across Child-Pugh subgroups: the GIDEON study. J Hepatol. 2016;65:1140–7. doi:10.1016/j.jhep.2016.07.020.
7. Geschwind J-F, Kudo M, Marrero JA, Venook AP, Chen X-P, Bronowicki J-P, et al. TACE treatment in patients with sorafenib-treated unresectable hepatocellular carcinoma in clinical practice: final analysis of GIDEON. Radiology. 2016;279:630–40. doi:10.1148/radiol.2015150667.
8. Wörns MA, Weinmann A, Pfingst K, Schulte-Sasse C, Messow C-M, Schulze-Bergkamen H, et al. Safety and efficacy of sorafenib in patients with advanced hepatocellular carcinoma in consideration of concomitant stage of liver cirrhosis. J Clin Gastroenterol. 2009;43:489–95. doi:10.1097/MCG.0b013e31818ddfc6.
9. Iavarone M, Cabibbo G, Piscaglia F, Zavaglia C, Grieco A, Villa E, et al. Field-practice study of sorafenib therapy for hepatocellular carcinoma: a prospective multicenter study in Italy. Hepatology. 2011;54:2055–63. doi:10.1002/hep.24644.
10. Varela M, Reig M, Álvarez-Navascués C, Forner A, Cadahía-Rodrigo V, Díaz A, González-Diéguez ML, Llarch N, Rodríguez M, Bruix J. La presencia de síntomas (performance status 0 vs 1) determina el pronóstico de los pacientes con carcinoma hepatocelular tratados con sorafenib. Asoc. Española para el Estud. las enfermedades Hepaticas; 2015.
11. Bruix J, Reig M, Sherman M. Evidence-based diagnosis, staging, and treatment of patients with hepatocellular carcinoma. Gastroenterology. 2016; doi:10.1053/j.gastro.2015.12.041.
12. Reig M, Gazzola A, Di Donato R, Bruix J. Systemic treatment. Best Pract Res Clin Gastroenterol. 2014;28:921–35. doi:10.1016/j.bpg.2014.08.003.
13. Di Costanzo GG, Tortora R, Iodice L, Lanza AG, Lampasi F, Tartaglione MT, et al. Safety and effectiveness of sorafenib in patients with hepatocellular carcinoma in clinical practice. Dig Liver Dis. 2012;44:788–92. doi:10.1016/j.dld.2012.04.001.
14. Vincenzi B, Santini D, Russo A, Addeo R, Giuliani F, Montella L, et al. Early skin toxicity as a predictive factor for tumor control in hepatocellular carcinoma patients treated with sorafenib. Oncologist. 2010;15:85–92. doi:10.1634/theoncologist.2009-0143.
15. Otsuka T, Eguchi Y, Kawazoe S, Yanagita K, Ario K, Kitahara K, et al. Skin toxicities and survival in advanced hepatocellular carcinoma patients treated with sorafenib. Hepatol Res. 2012;42:879–86. doi:10.1111/j.1872-034X.2012.00991.x.
16. Lee JH, Chung YH, Kim JA, Shim JH, Lee D, Lee HC, et al. Genetic predisposition of hand-foot skin reaction after sorafenib therapy in patients with hepatocellular carcinoma. Cancer. 2013;119:136–42. doi:10.1002/cncr.27705.
17. Reig M, Torres F, Rodriguez-Lope C, Forner A, LLarch N, Rimola J, et al. Early dermatologic adverse events predict better outcome in HCC patients treated with sorafenib. J Hepatol. 2014;61:318–24. doi:10.1016/j.jhep.2014.03.030.

18. Branco F, Saraiva R, Volt F, Sartori G, Kikuchi L, Chagas A, et al. The impact of early dermatologic events in the survival of patients with hepatocellular carcinoma treated with sorafenib. Ann Hepatol. 2017;16:263–8.
19. Palmer DH, Johnson PJ. Evaluating the role of treatment-related toxicities in the challenges facing targeted therapies for advanced hepatocellular carcinoma. Cancer Metastasis Rev. 2015;34:497–509. doi:10.1007/s10555-015-9580-2.
20. Llovet JM, Hernandez-Gea V. Hepatocellular carcinoma: reasons for phase III failure and novel perspectives on trial design. Clin Cancer Res. 2014;20:2072–9. doi:10.1158/1078-0432. CCR-13-0547.
21. Hollebecque A, Malka D, Ferté C, Ducreux M, Boige V. Systemic treatment of advanced hepatocellular carcinoma: from disillusions to new horizons. Eur J Cancer. 2015;51:327–39. doi:10.1016/j.ejca.2014.12.005.
22. Díaz-Gonzalez Á, Jordi R, Reig M, Darnell A, Varela M, Pons F, et al. Early dermatological adverse events and complete radiological response in Hcc patients treated with sorafenib. The link to treatment efficacy. ILCA 2015;ABSSUB-324.
23. Eltzschig HK, Carmeliet P. Hypoxia and inflammation. N Engl J Med. 2011;364:656–65. doi:10.1056/NEJMra0910283.
24. Nizet V, Johnson RS. Interdependence of hypoxic and innate immune responses. Nat Rev Immunol. 2009;9:609–17. doi:10.1038/nri2607.
25. Naugler WE, Karin M. NF-kappaB and cancer-identifying targets and mechanisms. Curr Opin Genet Dev. 2008;18:19–26. doi:10.1016/j.gde.2008.01.020.
26. Ponziani FR, Bhoori S, Germini A, Bongini M, Flores M, Sposito C, et al. Inducing tolerability of adverse events increases sorafenib exposure and optimizes patient's outcome in advanced hepatocellular carcinoma. Liver Int. 2015; doi:10.1111/liv.13052.
27. Therasse P, Arbuck SG, Eisenhauer EA, Wanders J, Kaplan RS, Rubinstein L, et al. New guidelines to evaluate the response to treatment in solid tumors. European Organization for Research and Treatment of Cancer, National Cancer Institute of the United States, National Cancer Institute of Canada. J Natl Cancer Inst. 2000;92:205–16.
28. Eisenhauer EA, Therasse P, Bogaerts J, Schwartz LH, Sargent D, Ford R, et al. New response evaluation criteria in solid tumours: revised RECIST guideline (version 1.1). Eur J Cancer. 2009;45:228–47. doi:10.1016/j.ejca.2008.10.026.
29. Reig M, Darnell A, Forner A, Rimola J, Ayuso C, Bruix J. Systemic therapy for hepatocellular carcinoma: the issue of treatment stage migration and registration of progression using the BCLC-refined RECIST. Semin Liver Dis. 2014;34:444–55. doi:10.1055/s-0034-1394143.
30. Lencioni R, Llovet J. Modified RECIST (mRECIST) assessment for hepatocellular carcinoma. Semin Liver Dis. 2010;30:052–60. doi:10.1055/s-0030-1247132.
31. Choi H, Charnsangavej C, Faria SC, Macapinlac HA, Burgess MA, Patel SR, et al. Correlation of computed tomography and positron emission tomography in patients with metastatic gastrointestinal stromal tumor treated at a single institution with imatinib mesylate: proposal of new computed tomography response criteria. J Clin Oncol. 2007;25:1753–9.
32. Ronot M, Bouattour M, Wassermann J, Bruno O, Dreyer C, Larroque B, et al. Alternative response criteria (Choi, European association for the study of the liver, and modified Response Evaluation Criteria in Solid Tumors [RECIST]) Versus RECIST 1.1 in patients with advanced hepatocellular carcinoma treated with sorafenib. Oncologist. 2014;19:394–402. doi:10.1634/theoncologist.2013-0114.
33. Gavanier M, Ayav A, Sellal C, Orry X, Claudon M, Bronowicki JP, et al. CT imaging findings in patients with advanced hepatocellular carcinoma treated with sorafenib: alternative response criteria (Choi, European Association for the Study of the Liver, and modified Response Evaluation Criteria in Solid Tumor (mRECIST)) versus. Eur J Radiol. 2016;85:103–12. doi:10.1016/j.ejrad.2015.10.024.
34. Bruix J, Sherman M, Llovet JM, Beaugrand M, Lencioni R, Burroughs AK, et al. Clinical management of hepatocellular carcinoma. Conclusions of the Barcelona-2000 EASL conference. European Association for the Study of the Liver. J Hepatol. 2001;35:421–30.

35. Huang L, Yoriko DS, Minghua S, Bruix J, Llovet J, Cheng A-L, et al. Weak correlation of overall survival and time to progression in advanced hepatocellular carcinoma. J Clin Oncol. 2017;35:(suppl 4S; abstract 23).
36. Iavarone M, Cabibbo G, Biolato M, Della Corte C, Maida M, Barbara M, et al. Predictors of survival of patients with advanced hepatocellular carcinoma who permanently discontinued sorafenib. Hepatology. 2015; doi:10.1002/hep.27729.
37. Ogasawara S, Chiba T, Ooka Y, Suzuki E, Kanogawa N, Saito T, et al. Post-progression survival in patients with advanced hepatocellular carcinoma resistant to sorafenib. Investig New Drugs. 2016;34:255–60. doi:10.1007/s10637-016-0323-1.
38. D'Amico G, Garcia-Tsao G, Pagliaro L. Natural history and prognostic indicators of survival in cirrhosis: a systematic review of 118 studies. J Hepatol. 2006;44:217–31. doi:10.1016/j.jhep.2005.10.013.
39. Tsochatzis EA, Bosch J, Burroughs AK. Future treatments of cirrhosis. Expert Rev Gastroenterol Hepatol. 2014;8:571–81. doi:10.1586/17474124.2014.902303.
40. Tsochatzis EA, Bosch J, Burroughs AK. Liver cirrhosis. Lancet. 2014;383:1749–61. doi:10.1016/S0140-6736(14)60121-5.
41. Cabibbo G, Enea M, Attanasio M, Bruix J, Craxi A, Camma C. A meta-analysis of survival rates of untreated patients in randomized clinical trials of hepatocellular carcinoma. Hepatology. 2010;51:1274–83. doi:10.1002/hep.23485.
42. Llovet JM, Bustamante J, Castells A, Vilana R, Ayuso Mdel C, Sala M, et al. Natural history of untreated nonsurgical hepatocellular carcinoma: rationale for the design and evaluation of therapeutic trials. Hepatology. 1999;29:62–7. doi:10.1002/hep.510290145.
43. Peer CJ, Sissung TM, Kim A, Jain L, Woo S, Gardner ER, et al. Sorafenib is an inhibitor of UGT1A1 but is metabolized by UGT1A9: implications of genetic variants on pharmacokinetics and hyperbilirubinemia. Clin Cancer Res. 2012;18:2099–107. doi:10.1158/1078-0432.CCR-11-2484.
44. Bruno S, Stroffolini T, Colombo M, Bollani S, Benvegnù L, Mazzella G, et al. Sustained virological response to interferon-alpha is associated with improved outcome in HCV-related cirrhosis: a retrospective study. Hepatology. 2007;45:579–87. doi:10.1002/hep.21492.
45. Reig M, Matilla A, Bustamante J, Castells L, de La Mata M, Delgado M, et al. Recommendations for the management of sorafenib in patients with hepatocellular carcinoma. Gastroenterol Hepatol. 2010;33:741–52. doi:10.1016/j.gastrohep.2010.05.007.
46. Bruix J, Sherman M. Management of hepatocellular carcinoma: an update. Hepatology. 2011;53:1020–2. doi:10.1002/hep.24199.
47. EASL-EORTC clinical practice guidelines: management of hepatocellular carcinoma. J Hepatol. 2012;56:908–43. doi:10.1016/j.jhep.2011.12.001.
48. Chen L-T, Liu T-W, Chao Y, Shiah H-S, Chang J-Y, Juang S-H, et al. alpha-fetoprotein response predicts survival benefits of thalidomide in advanced hepatocellular carcinoma. Aliment Pharmacol Ther. 2005;22:217–26. doi:10.1111/j.1365-2036.2005.02547.x.
49. Chan SL, Mo FKF, Johnson PJ, Hui EP, Ma BBY, Ho WM, et al. New utility of an old marker: serial alpha-fetoprotein measurement in predicting radiologic response and survival of patients with hepatocellular carcinoma undergoing systemic chemotherapy. J Clin Oncol. 2009;27:446–52. doi:10.1200/JCO.2008.18.8151.
50. Vora SR, Zheng H, Stadler ZK, Fuchs CS, Zhu AX. Serum alpha-fetoprotein response as a surrogate for clinical outcome in patients receiving systemic therapy for advanced hepatocellular carcinoma. Oncologist. 2009;14:717–25. doi:10.1634/theoncologist.2009-0038.
51. Shao Y-Y, Lin Z-Z, Hsu C, Shen Y-C, Hsu C-H, Cheng A-L. Early alpha-fetoprotein response predicts treatment efficacy of antiangiogenic systemic therapy in patients with advanced hepatocellular carcinoma. Cancer. 2010;116:4590–6. doi:10.1002/cncr.25257.
52. Kuzuya T, Asahina Y, Tsuchiya K, Tanaka K, Suzuki Y, Hoshioka T, et al. Early decrease in alpha-fetoprotein, but not des-gamma-carboxy prothrombin, predicts sorafenib efficacy in patients with advanced hepatocellular carcinoma. Oncology. 2011;81:251–8. doi:10.1159/000334454.
53. Yau T, Yao TJ, Chan P, Wong H, Pang R, Fan ST, et al. The significance of early alpha-fetoprotein level changes in predicting clinical and survival benefits in advanced hepatocel-

lular carcinoma patients receiving sorafenib. Oncologist. 2011;16(9):1270. doi:10.1634/theoncologist.2011-0105.

54. Kawaoka T, Aikata H, Murakami E, Nakahara T, Naeshiro N, Tanaka M, et al. Evaluation of the mRECIST and α-fetoprotein ratio for stratification of the prognosis of advanced-hepatocellular-carcinoma patients treated with sorafenib. Oncology. 2012;83:192–200. doi:10.1159/000341347.
55. Personeni N, Bozzarelli S, Pressiani T, Rimassa L, Tronconi MC, Sclafani F, et al. Usefulness of alpha-fetoprotein response in patients treated with sorafenib for advanced hepatocellular carcinoma. J Hepatol. 2012;57:101–7. doi:10.1016/j.jhep.2012.02.016.
56. Nakazawa T, Hidaka H, Takada J, Okuwaki Y, Tanaka Y, Watanabe M, et al. Early increase in α-fetoprotein for predicting unfavorable clinical outcomes in patients with advanced hepatocellular carcinoma treated with sorafenib. Eur J Gastroenterol Hepatol. 2013;25:683–9. doi:10.1097/MEG.0b013e32835d913b.
57. Varela M, Castaño-Fernández O, Garrido M, Blanco-García L, Martínez-Camblor P, Mesa-Álvarez A, et al. Time to progression of AFP (TPA) as a predictor of survival in hepatocellular carcinoma treated with sorafenib (SOR). J Cancer Ther. 2014;5:1332–43.
58. Kuzuya T, Ishigami M, Ishizu Y, Honda T, Hayashi K, Katano Y, et al. Early clinical response after 2 weeks of sorafenib therapy predicts outcomes and anti tumor response in patients with advanced hepatocellular carcinoma. PLoS One. 2015;10:e0138776. doi:10.1371/journal.pone.0138776.
59. Arrondeau J, Mir O, Boudou-Rouquette P, Coriat R, Ropert S, Dumas G, et al. Sorafenib exposure decreases over time in patients with hepatocellular carcinoma. Investig New Drugs. 2012;30:2046–9. doi:10.1007/s10637-011-9764-8.
60. Boudou-Rouquette P, Ropert S, Mir O, Coriat R, Billemont B, Tod M, et al. Variability of sorafenib toxicity and exposure over time: a pharmacokinetic/pharmacodynamic analysis. Oncologist. 2012;17:1204–12. doi:10.1634/theoncologist.2011-0439.
61. Boudou-Rouquette P, Narjoz C, Golmard JL, Thomas-Schoemann A, Mir O, Taieb F, et al. Early sorafenib-induced toxicity is associated with drug exposure and UGTIA9 genetic polymorphism in patients with solid tumors: a preliminary study. PLoS One. 2012;7:e42875. doi:10.1371/journal.pone.0042875PONE-D-12-07807.
62. Bins S, Lenting A, El Bouazzaoui S, van Doorn L, Oomen-de Hoop E, Eskens FA, et al. Polymorphisms in SLCO1B1 and UGT1A1 are associated with sorafenib-induced toxicity. Pharmacogenomics. 2016;17:1483–90. doi:10.2217/pgs-2016-0063.
63. Llovet JM, Pena CE, Lathia CD, Shan M, Meinhardt G, Bruix J. Plasma biomarkers as predictors of outcome in patients with advanced hepatocellular carcinoma. Clin Cancer Res. 2012;18:2290–300. doi:10.1158/1078-0432.CCR-11-2175.
64. Zhu AX, Park JO, Ryoo B-Y, Yen C-J, Poon R, Pastorelli D, et al. Ramucirumab versus placebo as second-line treatment in patients with advanced hepatocellular carcinoma following first-line therapy with sorafenib (REACH): a randomised, double-blind, multicentre, phase 3 trial. Lancet Oncol. 2015;16:859–70. doi:10.1016/S1470-2045(15)00050-9.
65. Swietach P, Hulikova A, Vaughan-Jones RD, Harris AL. New insights into the physiological role of carbonic anhydrase IX in tumour pH regulation. Oncogene. 2010;29:6509–21. doi:10.1038/onc.2010.455.
66. Reig M, Boix L, Forner A, Rodriguez de Lope C, Lopez-Oliva JM, Tremosini S, et al. Serum carbonic anhydrase 9 (CA) is a valuable biomarker (BM) to profile patients with hepatocellular carcinoma (HCC) treated with sorafenib and predict their outcome. J Heaptol 2011;Volume 54.
67. Reig M, Boix L, Torres F, Lopez-Oliva JM, Rimol J, Darnell A, et al. Optimization of survival prediction in patients under sorafenib treatmeent: usefulness of carbonic anhydrase IX baseline and baseline and evolutive angiopoyetin-2. J Hepatol. 2016;64
68. Bruix J, Qin S, Merle P, Granito A, Huang YH, Bodoky G, Pracht M, Yokosuka O, Rosmorduc O, Breder V, Gerolami R, Masi G, Ross PJ, Song T, Bronowicki JP, Ollivier-Hourmand I, Kudo M, Cheng AL, Llovet JM, Finn RS, LeBerre MA, Baumhauer A, Meinhardt G, Han G, RESORCE Investigators. Regorafenib for patients with hepatocellular carcinoma who progressed on sorafenib treatment (RESORCE): a randomised, double-blind, placebo-controlled, phase 3 trial. Lancet. 2017;389:56–66.

Overcoming Treatment Resistance in Hepatocellular Carcinoma: Regorafenib and Lessons from Other Malignancies

Bingnan Zhang and Richard S. Finn

Abstract This chapter will explore some of the known mechanisms mediating resistance in hepatocellular carcinoma (HCC). Despite the global burden of the disease, the treatment options for advanced HCC remain limited. Numerous studies have evaluated both single-agent and combination chemotherapy without any of these showing a definitive improvement in survival. The era of molecular targeted therapeutics ushered in great hope for the development of new and effective agents, however, for the past 10 years, only sorafenib has proven to be active against the disease. Only recently, has the multi-kinase inhibitor regorafenib now shown evidence of activity in the second-line setting. HCC has deservedly earned the title of a "resistant-tumor". The agents that have proven to be effective in so many other malignancies have failed which raises some of the unique biologic aspects of HCC, including the native chemical resistance mechanisms in hepatocytes given the liver's natural function in that area. The hope is that new molecular insights into HCC will provide a path forward for new effective treatments in advanced HCC. While there is precedent for this approach in other solid tumors, the strategy is yet to be exploited effectively in HCC.

Keywords Hepatocellular carcinoma • Targeted therapy • Resistance • Sorafenib • Regorafenib

B. Zhang
Department of Medicine, Division of Hematology/Oncology, Geffen School of Medicine, University of California, Los Angeles, Los Angeles, CA, USA

R.S. Finn (✉)
Department of Medicine, Division of Hematology/Oncology, Geffen School of Medicine, University of California, Los Angeles, Los Angeles, CA, USA

UCLA Translational Oncology,
2825 Santa Monica Blvd, Suite 200, Santa Monica, CA 90404, USA
e-mail: rfinn@mednet.ucla.edu

A. Villanueva (ed.), *Resistance to Molecular Therapies for Hepatocellular Carcinoma*, Resistance to Targeted Anti-Cancer Therapeutics,
DOI 10.1007/978-3-319-56197-4_8

Abbreviations

BCLC	Barcelona Clinic Liver Cancer
c-MET	Hepatocyte growth factor receptor
EGF	Epidermal growth factor
EMT	Epithelial-mesenchymal transition
FGF	Fibroblast growth factor
HCC	Hepatocellular carcinoma
HGF	Hepatocyte growth factor
IGF	Insulin growth factor
NASH	Non-alcoholic steatohepatitis
RTK	Receptor tyrosine kinases
TACE	Trans-arterial chemoembolization
TAE	Trans-arterial embolization
TGF-β	Transforming growth factor beta
VEGF	Vascular endothelial growth factor

Background

While the mortality of many common malignancies such as breast and colorectal cancer has been falling, hepatocellular carcinoma (HCC) remains one of the deadliest cancers with a rising mortality rate [1]. Unlike other tumor types, HCC has inherent challenges arising from its clinical and biologic complexity. For example, its tight association with underlying liver disease and cirrhosis represents a competing risk for death other than the tumor characteristics. Poor clinical trial designs that enrolled patients with severe liver dysfunction are likely responsible for some of the clinical failures to date [2]. More recently, the use of staging systems such as the BCLC which incorporate tumor characteristics as well as the performance status and the Child-Pugh score as an assessment of underlying liver function have corrected this flaw in trial design [3]. Still, even well conducted studies have not yielded robust clinical activity.

The natural history of HCC is such that even patients that are found with early and intermediate stage disease often recur after local treatments and eventually develop an advanced tumor stage characterized by invasion into the portal vasculature and extra-hepatic spread and declining performance status and liver function [4]. Drug development has concentrated on patients with these tumor characteristics [2]. By and large, the overwhelming majority of agents evaluated in HCC have been done so as an after-thought; drug "X" works in colon cancer so let's see if it works in liver cancer. This approach has not yielded clinical advances largely because it ignores the unique tumor biology of HCC and the likely inherent resistant mechanisms in HCC.

The Liver as a Toxin Resistant Organ

In normal anatomy, the liver receives the portal blood supply and serves to protect the systemic circulation from ingested toxins. As such several inherent mechanisms of toxin (i.e. drug) resistance exist in normal hepatocytes and are maintained in malignant cells. These include the expression of drug efflux pumps such as the p-glycoprotein family which remove toxins from the portal circulation for excretion the in bile [5]. It can be hypothesized that this characteristic alone may explain the difficulty in finding agents that are active in HCC.

Along a similar biologic rationale is the altered metabolism of drugs in the cirrhotic liver. Drug development in other tumor types often exclude patients with impaired liver function, whereas in the case of HCC, this is unavoidable. The diverse etiologies of HCC including hepatitis B and C, heavy alcohol use, diabetes and non-alcoholic steatohepatitis (NASH); or less commonly aflatoxin B1, hereditary hemochromatosis, α-1 antitrypsin deficiency, and autoimmune hepatitis all lead to liver inflammation, fibrosis, and cirrhosis which alter drug metabolism. The clinical complications of portal hypertension, platelet sequestration, varices and gastrointestinal bleeding, often limit the selection and adequate dosing of cytotoxic agents. In addition, alterations in intrinsic liver enzymes alter drug pharmacokinetics and metabolism which can greatly alter the exposure to these drugs [6].

The Failure of Cytotoxics

The backbone of cancer treatment for most tumors has been cytotoxic chemotherapy. In the context of HCC, this approach has failed. Local-regional use of various chemotherapy agents as part of trans-arterial chemoembolization (TACE) plays a key role in the management of intermediate HCC (i.e., BCLC stage B) but recent studies suggest that bland embolization (TAE), without chemotherapy is just as effective [7]. This observation challenges the hypotheses that a higher concentration of chemotherapy delivered directly to the tumor bed will overcome innate chemoresistance. The lack of proven efficacy of hepatic artery infused chemotherapy supports this idea as well.

Cytotoxic chemotherapies can generally be grouped by their mechanisms of action. These include antimetabolites, alkylating agents, microtubule poisons, platinum salts, anthracyclines, taxanes, and anti-tumor antibiotics. Numerous studies have evaluated these as single agents or in combination. The hypothesis behind combining agents with different mechanisms of action is that there will be synergy and an ability to overcome inherent resistance to any single agent/mechanism. While this approach often increased the response rates, a true survival advantage with any of these drugs has never been demonstrated. Regardless of this observation, until the approval of sorafenib in 2008, doxorubicin had been the de facto systemic treatment for advanced HCC (i.e., BCLC stage C). This was not based on

Table 1 Randomized trials of chemotherapy in HCC

Trial	Size (n)	Comparison	Result
Lai et al. [8]	106	Doxorubicin No treatment	OS: 10.6 v 7.5 wks *P* = 0.036
Yeo et al. [49]	188	PIAF Doxorubicin	OS: 8.7v 6.8 mos *P* = 0.83; HR, 0.97;95% CI = 0.71–1.32
Gish et al. [50]	445	Nolatrexed Doxorubicin	OS: 22.3 v 32.3 wks *P* = 0.0068; HR, 0.753
EACH [9]	371	FOLFOX-4 Doxorubicin	OS: 6.4 v 5.0 mos *P* = 0.07; HR, 0.80;95% CI, 0.63–1.02

PIAF platinum, interferon, adriamycin, 5-flurouracil, *OS* overall survival, *HR* hazard ratio, *CI* confidence interval, *mos* months, *wks* weeks

any strong clinical or scientific rationale. In fact, despite early studies that suggested increased toxicity from neutropenia and cardiotoxicity [8], doxorubicin was the control arm in several phase 3 chemotherapy based studies (Table 1). Recently, the EACH study assessed the safety and efficacy of oxaliplatin, 5-flurouracil, and leucovorin (FOLFOX-4 regimen) versus doxorubicin in a randomized study [9]. This study was a multicenter randomized Phase 2 study in Chinese patients with overall survival as the primary endpoint. While it did improve response rates, it did not improve overall survival. Based on the long history of cytotoxics in HCC, we can conclude that they are ineffective in treating HCC.

There are numerous molecular mechanisms that have been linked to resistance to specific cytotoxics in cancer. For example, amplification and/or increased activity of the dehydrofolate reductase (DHFR), the target for methrotrexate, has been shown to be a mechanism of resistance to methotrexate [10]; similarly, thymidylate synthetase expression and resistance to 5-flurouracil [11] and ERCC1 expression and sensitivity to platinum salts [12]. In general, these mechanisms are not validated and in practice are not used for patient selection.

Angiogenesis and HCC: Acquired and Innate Resistance

It has long been recognized that HCC is a hyper-vascular tumor and there is supportive evidence that alterations in the vascular endothelial growth factor (VEGF) pathway may be pathogenic in HCC [13]. There is now significant evidence that angiogenesis is important for tumor growth, invasion, and metastasis. Since 2000, there has been robust development of anti-angiogenics in cancer medicine, including monoclonal antibodies to VEGF (bevacizumab), the VEGF receptor (ramucirumab), and multiple small molecule tyrosine kinase inhibitors to the VEGF receptor (sorafenib, suntinib). In HCC, only sorafenib has been proven to extend survival in the first-line setting [14]. While sorafenib does have activity against the VEGF receptor, it has multiple other targets that may be important in HCC such as *raf* and

PDGFR as well [15]. With this in mind, the exact mechanism mediating sorafenib's anti-tumor activity in HCC is not known. An interesting laboratory study recently suggested that it is in the setting of HCC tumors that have amplification of the *VEGFA* gene that sorafenib mediates its effect by blocking VEGF-induced hepatocyte growth factor secretion from stromal cells, which then feeds-back and drives HCC cell growth [16]. Besides the clinical challenge of defining sorafenib resistance when the true response rate is close to zero, efforts to define molecular mechanisms of resistance have focused on overcoming resistance to anti-angiogenesis, and more recently other novel approaches.

There have been many concepts put forward about molecular mechanisms driving resistance to VEGF/R-directed therapies [17, 18]. These can be broken down into acquired and innate resistance. In regards to acquired resistance, this is in the setting of a tumor that initially had dependence on the VEGF-directed therapy and as a result induces a clinical response. Upregulation of bypass mechanisms for VEGF inhibition have been described such as fibroblast growth factor signaling and angiopoiten and ephrin-driven angiogenesis. These also include increased signaling through other receptor tyrosine kinases (RTKs) involved in tumor growth and proliferation such as the epidermal growth factor (EGF) or insulin growth factor (IGF). In addition, in the presence of VEGF blockade, the resulting hypoxia can induce the recruitment of bone marrow progenitor cells that can then induce angiogenesis independent of VEGF drivers [19]. Increased pericyte support of existing vasculature has also been described as an adaptive response to anti-angiogenic therapy as well as other mechanisms of invasion besides VEGF-induced [20].

Similarly, mechanisms of innate resistance have been described. More recently, the theory has emerged to explain intrinsic resistance to anti-angiogenic drugs by 'vessel co-option,' or the ability of tumors to hijack the existing vasculature in organs such as the lungs or liver, thus limiting the need for sprouting angiogenesis. Recent data suggest this may be a an additional mechanism for sorafenib resistance in HCC as well [21]. Pre-existing bypass mechanisms, such as alternative RTK signaling as mentioned above, or inflammatory cell protection of the vascular have been described.

The above mechanisms may be viewed as generic to anti-angiogenic therapy and may play a role in resistance to VEGF/R-directed therapy in HCC. However, given the clinical activity of sorafenib in HCC, there are several studies that have focused specifically on the question of sorafenib resistance. These have focused on tumor factors as well as stromal interactions. In reality, the clinical development has moved faster than our basic understanding of the molecular mechanisms underpinning sorafenib resistance. Many of the approaches come from hypotheses built in other malignancies, such as dual EGFR and VEGFR targeting in colon cancer [22] or the sequential use of anti-angiogenic agents in renal cell carcinoma [23]. These approaches have historically not yielded improvements in clinical outcomes.

Regorafenib as a Second-Line Therapy in Sorafenib-Resistant HCC: Next Steps

Molecular profiling studies of HCC tissue have identified that HCC is not "one disease" but distinct molecular subtypes [24, 25]. These reflect the cell of origin as well as acquired molecular alterations. Moving ahead, clinical studies are aiming to enrich patient populations for specific predictive markers, whether they are markers of a specific "subtype" of HCC, or specific genetic alterations. For example, there is evidence that suggests that TGF-β activation, a common alteration in HCC, is associated with the epithelial-mesenchymal transition (EMT) and is associated with sorafenib resistance [26, 27]. Similarly, Hedgehog signaling [28] and Wnt-pathway activation [29] have been associated with response to sorafenib as well. Figure 1 highlights many of the proposed mechanisms and targets for sorafenib resistance.

Regorafenib is an oral small molecule multikinase inhibitor that blocks activity of both wild-type and V599E mutant BRAF, as well as RTKs involved in angiogenesis including VEGFR-2,-3, platelet derived growth factor receptor beta, FLt-3, and c-KIT [30]. It was initially evaluated in single-arm phase 1 [31] and phase 2 [32, 33]

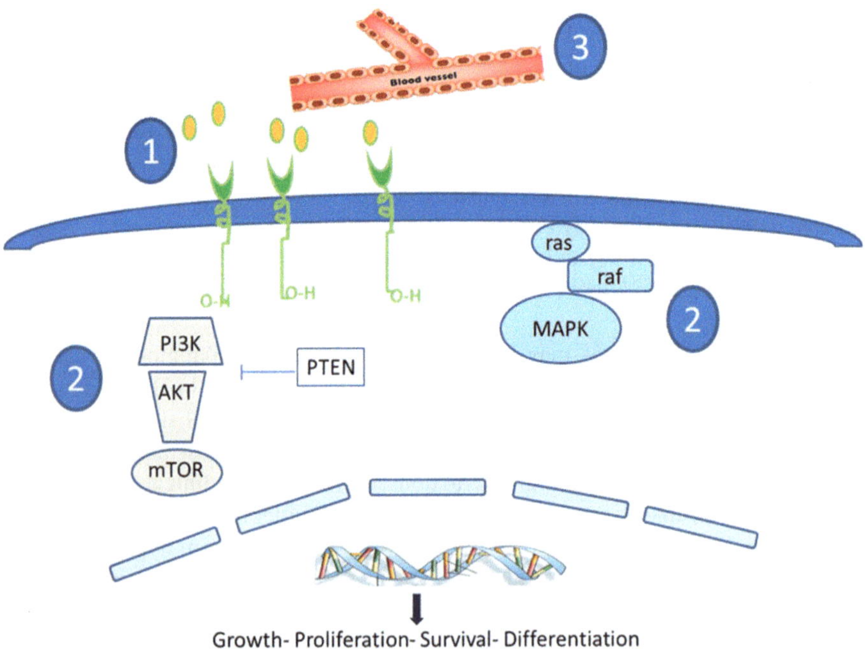

Fig. 1 Proposed mechanisms of sorafenib resistance. Sorafenib resistance has been associated with increased signaling through receptor tyrosine kinases (*1*), downstream intracellular signaling pathways such as the PI3K/AKT pathway (*2*), and alternative growth factors driving angiogenesis (*3*) such as cancer stem cells, among others

studies in patients with prior exposure to sorafenib. The safety profile was confirmed and there was evidence of tumor control. This led to the large randomized phase 3 RESORCE study which was the first study in nearly 10 years to demonstrate a survival advantage with a new systemic agent in HCC [32]. The results demonstrated a nearly 3-month improvement in overall survival with regorafenib in patients with documented progression on sorafenib. The safety and tolerability were acceptable and similar to those seen with sorafenib. This was accompanied by an improved response rate suggesting that despite its similarity to sorafenib, it is a different molecule with different molecular effects in HCC. While the exact mechanisms of action for regorafenib's clinical activity after sorafenib are unclear, there is precedent that the sequential use of multi-kinase inhibitors can improve clinical outcome, specifically, regorafenib has been shown to improve survival in patients with gastrointestinal stromal tumors after failure of prior multi-kinase inhibitors (imatinib and sunitnib) [34].

There have been several tumor mechanisms put forward as driving resistance to sorafenib in HCC. Increased expression and signaling through the hepatocyte growth factor receptor (HGFR/cMET) has been implicated in driving sorafenib resistance [35]. Increased expression of cMET has been described in tumors progressing on sorafenib [36]. Together these data have supported the phase 3 study evaluating the cMET inhibitor tivantinib in patients that have progressed on sorafenib. Patients in this study are pre-screened for increased c-MET expression by immunohistochemistry prior to enrollment. While this appraoch held promise, a press release in February 2017 stated that this study did not meet its primary endpoint of improving overall survival in MET-high patients. Besides tivantinib, there are newer MET inhibitors in early development as well [37]. Cabozantinib is a multi-kinase inhibitor with activity against cMET and other kinases currently being evaluated in a second-line setting for patients progressing on sorafenib though there is no biomarker being used to select patients

Other scientific observations that provide a mechanism for sorafenib resistance are generally in the pre-clinical phase or in early phase 1 and 2 clinical development [38]. In regards to tumor factors, alterations in intracellular signaling pathways have been implicated. Both hyper-activation of the PI3-kinase/AKT/mTOR [39, 40] and the *raf/ras*/MAP-kinase pathway [41] have been implicated. Increased signaling through both of these intracellular pathways can also occur from increased receptor tyrosine kinase signaling. In this regard, the epidermal growth factor receptor (EGFR) [42], insulin growth factor receptor (IGFR) [43–45], and fibroblast growth factor receptor (FGFR) [45, 46], and c-Met [47] mentioned above, all have some degree of laboratory rationale supporting their importance, though clinical data supporting that targeting these pathways improve outcomes are lacking.

Drawing from other malignancies, there is precedent for the rationale for biomarker trial designs to overcome resistance mechanisms. For example, in melanoma, about 60% are driven by the BRAF V600 mutation. Targeting the B-raf V600 mutant protein with the small molecule inhibitors vemurafenib or dabrefenib has been shown to improve survival in this selected population of patients. However, resistance to this approach has been shown to mediated by increased signaling in

RAF-MEK-ERK pathway (MAPK). To overcome this resistance, the MEK inhibitor trametinib has been studied as both a single agent and in combination with B-raf inhibitors. The resulting clinical study of the combination demonstrated a significant improvement in progression free-survival with combined B-raf and MEK inhibition. This example demonstrates the success of translating a biologic resistance mechanism into clinical practice [48]. As we increase our understanding of the molecular diversity of HCC and molecular drivers, this approach can impact trial designs in the future.

Conclusions

HCC is a difficult disease to treat. Not only because of its clinical association with underlying liver disease but its inherent resistance to therapies that have had significant activity in other tumor types. To date, the only systemic treatments that have proven efficacy are those with inexact mechanisms of action (sorafenib and regorafenib). Technology has allowed for a large increase in our knowledge of the molecular make-up of liver cancers, but still the clinical translation has been lacking. There are ongoing studies aimed at targeting specific mechanisms suggested to be important in mediating resistance to sorafenib, but perhaps even more important, are studies that are looking at targeting independent pathways in liver cancer, such as immune escape or populations of patients with specific genomic alterations. The recent results from the RESORCE study, after nearly 10 years of failed phase 3 studies, prove that we can improve outcomes for our patients but requires an ongoing commitment to basic and clinical research.

Conflict of Interest Dr. Richard S Finn has served as a consultant to Bayer, Pfizer, Novartis, Bristol Myers Squibb, Eisai.

References

1. Siegel RL, Miller KD, Jemal A. Cancer statistics, 2016. CA Cancer J Clin. 2016;66:7–30.
2. Llovet JM, Di Bisceglie AM, Bruix J, et al. Design and endpoints of clinical trials in hepatocellular carcinoma. J Natl Cancer Inst. 2008;100:698–711.
3. Bruix J, Reig M, Sherman M. Evidence-based diagnosis, staging, and treatment of patients with hepatocellular carcinoma. Gastroenterology. 2016;150:835–53.
4. Finn RS. Treatment of intermediate-stage hepatocellular carcinoma. Gastroenterol Hepatol. 2015;11:545–7.
5. Choi YH, Yu AM. ABC transporters in multidrug resistance and pharmacokinetics, and strategies for drug development. Curr Pharm Des. 2014;20:793–807.
6. Pinter M, Trauner M, Peck-Radosavljevic M, Sieghart W. Cancer and liver cirrhosis: implications on prognosis and management. ESMO Open. 2016;1:e000042.
7. Facciorusso A, Serviddio G, Muscatiello N. Transarterial radioembolization vs chemoembolization for hepatocarcinoma patients: a systematic review and meta-analysis. World J Hepatol. 2016;8:770–8.

8. Lai CL, Wu PC, Chan GC, Lok AS, Lin HJ. Doxorubicin versus no antitumor therapy in inoperable hepatocellular carcinoma. A prospective randomized trial. Cancer. 1988;62:479–83.
9. Qin S, Bai Y, Lim HY, et al. Randomized, multicenter, open-label study of oxaliplatin plus fluorouracil/leucovorin versus doxorubicin as palliative chemotherapy in patients with advanced hepatocellular carcinoma from Asia. J Clin Oncol. 2013;31:3501–8.
10. Bertino JR, Goker E, Gorlick R, Li WW, Banerjee D. Resistance mechanisms to methotrexate in tumors. Oncologist. 1996;1:223–6.
11. Peters GJ, Backus HH, Freemantle S, et al. Induction of thymidylate synthase as a 5-fluorouracil resistance mechanism. Biochim Biophys Acta. 2002;1587:194–205.
12. Martin LP, Hamilton TC, Schilder RJ. Platinum resistance: the role of DNA repair pathways. Clin Cancer Res. 2008;14(5):1291.
13. Finn RS, Zhu AX. Targeting angiogenesis in hepatocellular carcinoma: focus on VEGF and bevacizumab. Expert Rev Anticancer Ther. 2009;9:503–9.
14. Llovet JM, Ricci S, Mazzaferro V, et al. Sorafenib in advanced hepatocellular carcinoma. N Engl J Med. 2008;359:378–90.
15. Wilhelm SM, Adnane L, Newell P, Villanueva A, Llovet JM, Lynch M. Preclinical overview of sorafenib, a multikinase inhibitor that targets both Raf and VEGF and PDGF receptor tyrosine kinase signaling. Mol Cancer Ther. 2008;7:3129–40.
16. Horwitz E, Stein I, Andreozzi M, et al. Human and mouse VEGFA-amplified hepatocellular carcinomas are highly sensitive to sorafenib treatment. Cancer Discov. 2014;4:730–43.
17. Weis SM, Cheresh DA. Tumor angiogenesis: molecular pathways and therapeutic targets. Nat Med. 2011;17:1359–70.
18. Bergers G, Hanahan D. Modes of resistance to anti-angiogenic therapy. Nat Rev Cancer. 2008;8:592–603.
19. Ellis LM, Hicklin DJ. Pathways mediating resistance to vascular endothelial growth factor-targeted therapy. Clin Cancer Res. 2008;14:6371–5.
20. Niu G, Chen X. Vascular endothelial growth factor as an anti-angiogenic target for cancer therapy. Curr Drug Targets. 2010;11:1000–17.
21. Kuczynski EA, Kerbel RS. Implications of vessel co-option in sorafenib-resistant hepatocellular carcinoma. Chin J Cancer. 2016;35:97.
22. Hecht JR, Mitchell E, Chidiac T, et al. A randomized phase IIIB trial of chemotherapy, bevacizumab, and panitumumab compared with chemotherapy and bevacizumab alone for metastatic colorectal cancer. J Clin Oncol. 2009;27:672–80.
23. Cohen RB, Oudard S. Antiangiogenic therapy for advanced renal cell carcinoma: management of treatment-related toxicities. Investig New Drugs. 2012;30:2066–79.
24. Lee JS, Heo J, Libbrecht L, et al. A novel prognostic subtype of human hepatocellular carcinoma derived from hepatic progenitor cells. Nat Med. 2006;12:410–6.
25. Zucman-Rossi J, Villanueva A, Nault JC, Llovet JM. Genetic landscape and biomarkers of hepatocellular carcinoma. Gastroenterology. 2015;149:1226–39. e4
26. Fernando J, Malfettone A, Cepeda EB, et al. A mesenchymal-like phenotype and expression of CD44 predict lack of apoptotic response to sorafenib in liver tumor cells. Int J Cancer. 2015;136:E161–72.
27. Xin HW, Ambe CM, Miller TC, et al. Liver label retaining cancer cells are relatively resistant to the reported anti-cancer stem cell drug metformin. J Cancer. 2016;7:1142–51.
28. Chen X, Lingala S, Khoobyari S, Nolta J, Zern MA, Wu J. Epithelial mesenchymal transition and hedgehog signaling activation are associated with chemoresistance and invasion of hepatoma subpopulations. J Hepatol. 2011;55:838–45.
29. Lachenmayer A, Alsinet C, Savic R, et al. Wnt-pathway activation in two molecular classes of hepatocellular carcinoma and experimental modulation by sorafenib. Clin Cancer Res. 2012;18:4997–5007.
30. Wilhelm SM, Carter C, Tang L, et al. BAY 43-9006 exhibits broad spectrum oral antitumor activity and targets the RAF/MEK/ERK pathway and receptor tyrosine kinases involved in tumor progression and angiogenesis. Cancer Res. 2004;64:7099–109.

31. Finn RS, Blumenschein GR, Tolcher AW, Leong S, Boix O, Diefenbach K. Continuous-dose regorafenib (REG) in hepatocellular carcinoma (HCC): phase I safety and pharmacokinetic (PK) study. ASCO GI Symposium 2013; Abstract 300.
32. Bruix J, Qin S, Merle P, Granito A, et al. Regorafenib for patients with hepatocellular carcinoma who progressed on sorafenib treatment (RESORCE): a randomised, double-blind, placebo-controlled, phase 3 trial. Lancet. 2017;389:56–66.
33. Bruix J, Tak WY, Gasbarrini A, et al. Regorafenib as second-line therapy for intermediate or advanced hepatocellular carcinoma: multicentre, open-label, phase II safety study. Eur J Cancer. 2013;49:3412–9.
34. Demetri GD, Reichardt P, Kang YK, et al. Efficacy and safety of regorafenib for advanced gastrointestinal stromal tumours after failure of imatinib and sunitinib (GRID): an international, multicentre, randomised, placebo-controlled, phase 3 trial. Lancet. 2013;381:295–302.
35. Santoro A, Rimassa L, Borbath I, et al. Tivantinib for second-line treatment of advanced hepatocellular carcinoma: a randomised, placebo-controlled phase 2 study. Lancet Oncol. 2013;14:55–63.
36. Rimassa L, Abbadessa G, Personeni N, Port C, Borbath I, et al. Tumor and plasma biomarker analysis from the randomized controlled phase 2 trial of tivantinib in second-line hepatocellular carcinoma. ASCO GI Symposium 2016; Asbtract 197.
37. Zhang B, Finn RS. Personalized clinical trials in hepatocellular carcinoma based on biomarker selection. Liver Cancer. 2016;5:221–32.
38. Nishida N, Kitano M, Sakurai T, Kudo M. Molecular mechanism and prediction of sorafenib chemoresistance in human hepatocellular carcinoma. Dig Dis. 2015;33:771–9.
39. Villanueva A, Chiang DY, Newell P, et al. Pivotal role of mTOR signaling in hepatocellular carcinoma. Gastroenterology. 2008;135:1972–83, 1983.e1–11.
40. Finn RS, Poon RT, Yau T, et al. Phase I study investigating everolimus combined with sorafenib in patients with advanced hepatocellular carcinoma. J Hepatol. 2013;59:1271–7.
41. Rudalska R, Dauch D, Longerich T, et al. In vivo RNAi screening identifies a mechanism of sorafenib resistance in liver cancer. Nat Med. 2014;20:1138–46.
42. Blivet-Van Eggelpoel MJ, Chettouh H, Fartoux L, et al. Epidermal growth factor receptor and HER-3 restrict cell response to sorafenib in hepatocellular carcinoma cells. J Hepatol. 2012;57:108–15.
43. Tovar V, Cornella H, Moeini A, et al. Tumour initiating cells and IGF/FGF signalling contribute to sorafenib resistance in hepatocellular carcinoma. Gut. 2017;66:530–40.
44. Xu Y, Huang J, Ma L, et al. MicroRNA-122 confers sorafenib resistance to hepatocellular carcinoma cells by targeting IGF-1R to regulate RAS/RAF/ERK signaling pathways. Cancer Lett. 2016;371:171–81.
45. Tai WT, Cheng AL, Shiau CW, et al. Dovitinib induces apoptosis and overcomes sorafenib resistance in hepatocellular carcinoma through SHP-1-mediated inhibition of STAT3. Mol Cancer Ther. 2012;11:452–63.
46. Finn RS, Kang YK, Mulcahy M, et al. Phase II, open-label study of brivanib as second-line therapy in patients with advanced hepatocellular carcinoma. Clin Cancer Res. 2012;18:2090–8.
47. Xiao GH, Jeffers M, Bellacosa A, Mitsuuchi Y, Vande Woude GF, Testa JR. Anti-apoptotic signaling by hepatocyte growth factor/Met via the phosphatidylinositol 3-kinase/Akt and mitogen-activated protein kinase pathways. Proc Natl Acad Sci U S A. 2001;98:247–52.
48. Long GV, Stroyakovskiy D, Gogas H, et al. Combined BRAF and MEK inhibition versus BRAF inhibition alone in melanoma. N Engl J Med. 2014;371:1877–88.
49. Yeo W, Mok TS, Zee B, et al. A randomized phase III study of doxorubicin versus cisplatin/interferon alpha-2b/doxorubicin/fluorouracil (PIAF) combination chemotherapy for unresectable hepatocellular carcinoma. J Natl Cancer Inst. 2005;97:1532–8.
50. Gish RG, Porta C, Lazar L, et al. Phase III randomized controlled trial comparing the survival of patients with unresectable hepatocellular carcinoma treated with nolatrexed or doxorubicin. J Clin Oncol. 2007;25:3069–75.

Index

A. Villanueva (ed.), *Resistance to Molecular Therapies for Hepatocellular Carcinoma*, Resistance to Targeted Anti-Cancer Therapeutics,
DOI 10.1007/978-3-319-56197-4

MIX
Papier aus verantwortungsvollen Quellen
Paper from responsible sources
FSC® C105338

If you have any concerns about our products,
you can contact us on
ProductSafety@springernature.com

In case Publisher is established outside the EU,
the EU authorized representative is:
Springer Nature Customer Service Center GmbH
Europaplatz 3, 69115 Heidelberg, Germany

Printed by Libri Plureos GmbH
in Hamburg, Germany